Maat Philosophy vs. Fascism and the Police State

Volume II

MAAT PHILOSOPHY
vs.
Fascism,
The Police State,
Totalitarianism,
Great Reset, Covid 19,
Medical Tyranny,
Neo-Feudalism
and
the Path to
Political
&
Spiritual Freedom

Sema Institute/Cruzian Mystic Books
P.O.Box 570459
Miami, Florida, 33257
(305) 378-6253 Fax: (305) 378-6253

First U.S. edition © 2021 By Reginald Muata Ashby

All rights reserved. No part of this book may be used or reproduced in any manner whatsoever without written permission (address above) except in the case of brief quotations embodied in critical articles and reviews. All inquiries may be addressed to the address above.

The author is available for group lectures and individual counseling. For further information contact the publisher.

Ashby, Muata
Maat Philosophy vs Fascism and the Police State Vol. 2
ISBN: 9781937016739

Library of Congress Cataloging in Publication Data

Other books by Muata Ashby

See catalog in the back section for more listings

Table of Contents

PREFACE 7

Who is Maat? Maat as a Spiritual Philosophy............................ 10

Reflection 13

INTRODUCTION 14

Confronting the Issues of Life to Resolve Social Pathologies and Social Prosperity 15

Economic Malfeasance and Political Corruption in the year 2020 17

IMF heightens warnings on corporate debt following central bank cuts. 17

Who are the power elites?... 18

How the Power Elite Exercise their Power 21

The Power Elite Plan for Economic Devastation, Social Destruction and Remaking 22

The year 2020 revealed Fascism and the Police State in ascendancy... 27

Lies, facemasks, social distancing, and lockdowns 31

Safe and effective drug and supplement alternatives to vaccines ignored and denied by Health Officials with support from mainstream media-despite the proofs of their efficacy............................. 47

Tools for coercive psychological conditioning and the willingness to use them 48

Presidents, prime ministers as lightning rods to distract populations. 56

Medical Tyranny as a tool of the Power Elites......................... 58

Fear Appeal as a tool of sociopathic power elite tyrants 60

Fear Appeal and The "New Normal" meme............................. 62

The Fraud of Vaccines and Vaccines as tools of the power elites, medical tyranny and profits 65

Fraudulent Death tolls as a tool for supporting the Fear Appeal...... 67

Implications so far 71

Change in how cycle thresholds are manipulated in the PCR tests to produce the desired number of "cases" sufficient to scare the population and justify medical tyranny... 71

Sweden Says PCR Tests "Cannot Be Used To Determine Whether Someone Is Contagious" 73

- Reflections.. 74
  - More Examples of the Corruptions revealed in the year 2020......... 76

Democrat Party vs. Republican Party politics in the response to corona virus disease (covid 19) 79

- The fallacy of excess mortality due to corona virus 82
- Covidiocy or Covidmania 83

The Corruption of the CDC and the dubious corona virus so-called vaccines 85

Self-Delusion, Disempowerment, Spiritual bankruptcy and Political Enslavement.. 87

- The delusion (incapacity and or unwillingness to face the truth of) of race and racism... 88
- The delusion (incapacity and or unwillingness to face the truth of) of terrorist vs. the good guy. 89
- From Feudalism to Neo-feudalism 94
- The delusion (incapacity and or unwillingness to face the truth) of terror vs. security and humanitarianism. 97

Fauci Admits Wearing A Mask While Fully Vaccinated Was Political Theater 98

- The delusion (incapacity and or unwillingness to face the truth of) of democracy vs. fascism. 99
- The delusion about capitalism versus equal opportunity. 100

Political intolerance, "Woke culture", "MeeToo", "Millennial Fragility" and "cancel culture" blossoming into full blown corporate and government endorsed censorship. 101

- CURRENT DAY COMMON EXAMPLES OF POWER ELITE FASCISM IN THE USA and ABROAD: 106

- Capitalism, Fascism and the illusion of democracy 117

  - USA Government designed for tyranny of the minority over the majority.. 122

  - The Purposeful Failure of Trickle-down economics, lower interest rates, and bail-outs that enrich the power elites and impoverish everyone else.. 127

  - The Coronavirus and the global plan of domination by the power elites 134

  - From Lockdowns to vaccine passports to coerced vaccinations. 144

  - Protests and Socio-political-economic Change 150

- The Dire Prospects for the Future of Human Society and the Challenges Ahead for Successful Spiritual Life and Working Towards a Better World 155

  - TWO POWER ELITE SPONSORED GREAT RESETS FACING THE WORLD POPULATIONS 156

    - Medical Martial law and Medical emergencies as tools to allow the power elite to usher in totalitarianism.. 157

    - THE FRAUD OF VACCINE EFFICACY 161

- Looking Ahead: 2021 and beyond 169

  - From Barbarians to Snowflakes: Sociopathy, Fragility, Fear and Social Degradation.. 172

  - The Bane of Humanity and the answer from Ethiocracy 176

    - The Failure of the US constitution and the Delusion of the Founding Fathers 176

    - Ancient Egyptian Wisdom of Secular Government 176

    - Personal Sovereignty as a foundation for Secular Social Balance and Prosperity and Spiritual Enlightenment 177

- CONCLUSION: A Spiritual Appeal from Ancient Egyptian Maat Wisdom 178

  - The austerity of MAAT means… 180

INDEX 186

Other Books From C M Books 191

PREFACE

ANCIENT EGYPTIAN PROVERBS ON MAAT PHILOSOPHY

"When opulence and extravagance are a necessity instead of righteousness and truth, society will be governed by greed and injustice."

"When emotions are societies objective, tyranny will govern regardless of the ruling class."

"MAAT is great and its effectiveness lasting; it has not been disturbed since the time of Osiris. There is punishment for those who pass over its laws, but this is unfamiliar to the covetous one....When the end is nigh, *MAAT* lasts."

"Those who live today will die tomorrow, those who die tomorrow will be born again; Those who live MAAT will not die."

"No one reaches the beneficent West (heaven) unless their heart is righteous by doing *MAAT*. There is no distinction made between the inferior and the superior person; it only matters that one is found faultless when the balances and the two weights stand before the Lord of Eternity. No one is free from the reckoning. Thoth, a baboon, holds the balances to count each one according to what they have done upon earth."

"The sky is at peace, the earth is in joy, for they have heard that the King will set right the place of disorder. Tutankhamon drove out disorder from the Two Lands, and *MAAT* is firmly established in its place; he made lying an abomination, and the land is as it was at the first time."

"Speak *MAAT*; do *MAAT*."

"They who revere *MAAT* are *long-lived*; they who are covetous have no tomb."

"Do *MAAT* for the King, for *MAAT* is that which God loves! Speak *MAAT* to the King for that which the King loves is *MAAT!*"

Doing Maat is breath to the nose.

I am pure. I am pure. I am Pure.

I have washed my front parts with the waters of libations, I have cleansed my hinder parts with drugs which make wholly clean, and my inward parts have been washed in the liquor of Maat.

The Scribe Nu

Above: The Feather of Maat
Symbol of Truth, Righteousness, Justice and Social Order

The Philosophy of Maat is perhaps the oldest known philosophy of ethics and righteous action which when followed and understood proficiently, leads to spiritual evolution in the individual human being as well as the society which practices it. Originating in ancient Egypt before 5,500 BCE, the philosophy of MAAT is symbolized by a goddess who is the daughter of the Supreme Being (Ra), creator of the Cosmos. MAAT herself is "the foundation of the Cosmos" and MAAT symbolizes Truth, Justice, Order, Regularity, etc. Therefore, those who live a life based on truth, that is, with these virtues, will come into harmony with MAAT and thus the Universe itself and thereby with God as well. In this harmony, true happiness is to be found. Those who act in discord with MAAT, that is, those who live unrighteously and in disharmony with nature (termed neteru -divine cosmic forces) will suffer the consequences of their actions as dictated by the law of a cause and effect (Meskhenet - Karma). They will be subject to experience the judgment of their un-righteous actions from their own Higher Self.

For students of African Culture and Philosophy, the concept of Maat has engendered a renewed interest in Africa as a birthplace of ideas and philosophy. Having its origin in the Ancient Egyptian Wisdom Texts, Maat Philosophy encompasses disciplines and injunctions of virtuous living for promoting social order and peace at the level of individual human beings, families, communities, societies, and as a humanity. Thus, it is a universal concept of life, applicable to all. Maat was the epitome of social order which allowed Ancient Egyptian society to persist in harmony for THOUSANDS OF YEARS. Maat Philosophy is the concept that righteousness and truth must be the focus of every aspect of society (including government, religious institutions, and educational institutions). Maat was viewed as the basis for marriage and all relations. The Sages who created it saw the pitfalls of sexism, racism, greed, and other social evils and they understood that when people act in harmony with nature and in truth, their relations and mental dispositions are harmonious. This promotes order and peace in society and this allows society to persist and evolve in a positive manner. The understanding is that without righteousness and truth, i.e. ethical conscience, nothing of higher value can really be accomplished. In this sense, even great material accomplishments and achievements in society are of lesser value because they will not fulfill human beings who are not righteous.

Thus, Maat was seen as a Secular and well as a Non-secular discipline to be applied to all members of society. This ideal is held to be most beneficial throughout ancient Africa and it found its greatest expression in Ancient Egyptian culture. In early times, Maat was seen as a universal philosophy of life, akin to Confucianism. In later times Maat was depicted as a feather and as a goddess of justice, righteousness, and order. So Maat Philosophy developed from a philosophy of righteousness and social order to an association with a spiritual goal of life. These images were adopted by the Greeks and Romans who came to Egypt to study the philosophy. (See the book *From Egypt to Greece)*. Thus, Western culture was influenced early on by Maat Philosophy and its influences continue to be evident even at present.

WHO IS MAAT? MAAT AS A SPIRITUAL PHILOSOPHY

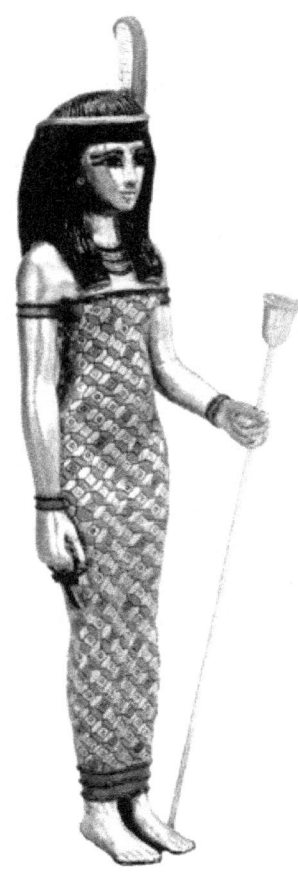

MAAT is the *daughter of Ra,* and she was with him on His celestial boat when he first emerged from the primeval waters along with His Company of gods and goddesses. She is also known as the *eye of Ra, lady of heaven, queen of the earth, mistress of the Netherworld, and the lady of the gods and goddesses.* MAAT also has a dual form or *MAATI.* In her *capacity* of God, MAAT is *Shes MAAT* which means *ceaselessness and regularity* of the course of the sun (i.e. the universe). In the form of MAATI, she represents the South and the North which symbolize Upper and Lower Egypt as well as the Higher and Lower Self. MAAT is the personification of justice and righteousness upon which God has created the universe and MAAT is also the essence of God and creation. Therefore, it is MAAT who judges the soul when it arrives in the judgment hall of MAAT. Sometimes MAAT herself becomes the scales upon which the heart of the initiate is judged. MAAT judges the heart (unconscious mind) of the initiate in an attempt to determine to what extent the heart has lived in accordance with MAAT or truth, correctness, reality, genuineness, uprightness, righteousness, justice, steadfastness, and the unalterable order of creation.

The ancient Egyptian Goddess MAAT holds a papyrus reed scepter. Papyrus is the ancient medium or writing upon which the teachings of wisdom are recorded. She is the symbolic embodiment of world order, justice, righteousness, correctness, harmony, and peace. She is also known by her headdress composed of a feather of truth. Her name is synonymous with mother since the syllable *"ma"* is a universal hekau or mantram signifying mother in many countries of the world. For example, mother in English, madre in Spanish, mata in Hindi all convey the same meaning. All of these arise from the root *Ma.* Thus, she is also known as *Ma* or *Maa* or the universal mother, the cosmic mother. She is a form of the Goddess Isis, *Aset/Auset,* who represents wisdom and spiritual awakening.

When Ra emerged in his Boat for the first time and brought creation into being, he was standing on the pedestal of Maat. Thus the Creator, Ra, lives by Maat and has established Creation on Maat. Who is Maat? Maat represents the very order which constitutes creation. Therefore, it is said that Ra created the universe by putting Maat in the place of chaos. So creation itself is Maat. Creation without order is chaos. Maat is a profound teaching about the nature of creation and the manner in which human conduct should be cultivated in order to experience order and truth instead of chaos. It refers to a deep understanding of Divinity and how virtuous qualities can be developed in the human heart so as to come closer to the Divine.

So, again, Maat is a philosophy, a spiritual symbol as well as cosmic energy or force which pervades the entire universe. She is the symbolic embodiment of world order, justice, righteousness, correctness, harmony, and peace. She is also known by her headdress composed of a feather of truth.

In ancient Egypt, the judges and all those connected with the judicial system were initiated into the teachings of MAAT. Thus, those who would discharge the laws and regulations of society were well trained in the ethical and spiritual-mystical values of life (presented in this volume), fairness, justice, and the responsibility to serve society in order to promote harmony in society and the possibility for spiritual development in an atmosphere of freedom and peace. Only when there is justice and fairness in society can there be an abiding harmony and peace. Harmony and peace are necessary for the pursuit of true happiness and inner fulfillment in life.

Along with her associates, the goddesses *Shai, Rennenet,* and *Meskhenet*, Maat encompass the teachings known in modern times as Karma and Reincarnation, or the destiny of every individual based on past actions, thoughts, and feelings. Thus, they have an important role to play in the Judgment scene of the Book of Coming Forth By Day. Understanding their principles leads the aspirant to become free of the cycle of reincarnation and human suffering and to discover supreme bliss and immortality.

MAAT signifies *that which is straight*. Two of the symbols of MAAT are the ostrich feather (𓆄) and the pedestal (▭) upon which God stands. The Supreme Being, in the form of the God *Ptah,* is one of the Divinities often depicted standing on the pedestal.

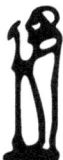

MAAT is the daughter of Ra, the high God, thus in a hymn to Ra we find:

> *The land of Manu* (the West) *receives thee with satisfaction, and the goddess MAAT embraces thee both at morn and at eve... the god Djehuty and the goddess MAAT have written down thy daily course for thee every day...*

Another Hymn in the Papyrus of Qenna provides deeper insight into MAAT. Qenna says:

> *I have come to thee, O Lord of the Gods, Temu-Heru-khuti, whom MAAT directeth... Amen-Ra rests upon MAAT... Ra lives by MAAT... Osiris carries along the earth in His train by MAAT...*

MAAT is the *daughter of Ra,* and she was with him on His celestial boat when he first emerged from the primeval waters along with His Company of gods and goddesses. She is also known as the *Eye of Ra, lady of heaven, queen of the earth, mistress of the Underworld, and the lady of the gods and goddesses.* MAAT also has a dual form or *MAATI.* In her *capacity* of God, MAAT is *Shes MAAT* which means *ceaselessness and regularity* of the course of the sun (i.e. the universe). In the form of MAATI (dual truth), she represents the South and the North which symbolize Upper and Lower Egypt as well as the Higher and Lower Self. MAAT is the personification of justice and righteousness upon which God has created the universe and MAAT is also the essence of God manifested as creation. Therefore, it is MAAT who judges the soul when it arrives in the judgment hall of MAAT. Sometimes MAAT herself becomes the scales upon which the heart of the initiate is judged. MAAT judges the heart (unconscious mind) of the initiate in an attempt to determine to what extent the heart has lived in accordance with MAAT or truth, correctness, reality, genuineness, uprightness, righteousness, justice, steadfastness, and the unalterable nature of creation.

REFLECTION

Present-day society is at a crossroads manifesting as a struggle between Maat, what is true, righteous, balanced, and orderly, against the designs for a power elite controlling world politics and economics bent on control, power, and genocide. This book is a continuing chronicling of the ethical deviations of society but also a solution-seeking journey in service of the higher nature of humanity as expressed in the Ancient Egyptian wisdom and spiritual philosophy of MAAT, which is the ethical conscience legacy for all humanity.

INTRODUCTION

This is an update to the book *Maat vs. Fascism and the Police State* (2014) and a warning about the fast-evolving nature of the breakdown of USA society, economics, and politics.

In the Fall of the year 2019 something momentous occurred. In that year there was a collapse of the Bank Repo market, which was a continuation of the banking system crash of 2008 that was facilitated by the Federal Reserve central bank and the politicians, which was responded to, this time (2020), by the US central bank, the Federal Reserve, in a similar way, with zero interest rate policy and perpetual bailouts, that is, pouring newly created currency, out of thin air (bank counterfeiting), into the banking system to temporarily prevent an economic collapse, similar to or worse than the one during the 2008-2009 economic crisis. As the banking crisis restarted in the fall of 2019, the International Monetary Fund warned that corporate debt could be at risk in another global downturn. The major downturn began in 2020 in the midst of zero interest rate policy and perpetual bailouts, for the benefit of corporations. As allowed by the government regulatory authorities, corporations ignored any cautions and continued accumulating debt to increase profits which made them and the society financially vulnerable due to the malfeasance.

In response to a supposed pandemic, untested and unscientific society-wide lockdowns were imposed. Businesses that could not survive the imposed lockdowns, some 40-70%, were/are entering into bankruptcy and closing for good. This state of affairs is a faster downturn than the Great Depression of the 1930s. The result of the depression of the 1930s included:[1]

- ✓ Effects of the Great Depression:[2]
- ✓ 20% of the population was unemployed
- ✓ Suicide rose to an all-time high in the United States
- ✓ Two million men and women became traveling hobos (homeless)
- ✓ 273,000 lost their homes
- ✓ Unemployment in Europe averaged 20%

---

[1] https://youtu.be/gOkaQPmftXg
[2] www.history.com/news/life-for-the-average-family-during-the-great-depression

- ✓ 25% of the U.S. workforce was unemployed
- ✓ Even upper-middle class professionals, such as doctors and lawyers, saw their incomes drop by as much as 40 percent.

In the year 2020-2021, a supposedly new virus began to affect a part of the human population. The term "supposedly" is used because many questions emerged about the origins and true severity of the disease, which have not been resolved. In response, to the disease, in a coordinated fashion, without scientific evidence or logic, governments around the world imposed lockdowns that shut down most of the economies of those countries. Yet, corporations and politicians remained in denial, or purposely ignored the situation; consequently, the population at large, unsuspecting, is going along with the propaganda from politicians, the banks, and the media about the supposedly good state of the economy.

The Next Global Depression is Coming and Optimism Won't Slow it Down
August 6, 2020[3]

CONFRONTING THE ISSUES OF LIFE TO RESOLVE SOCIAL PATHOLOGIES AND SOCIAL PROSPERITY

This book specifically treats the issue of social, political, economic, and medical ethics surrounding how the leaders of the society have acted about their charge of protecting the wellbeing of the population. In reference to the part of the medical ethics of this volume, this deals with the disease that has been named "covid 19". This author does not deny that *there is indeed a "disease process"* that has affected especially those who are elderly and who have co-morbid health conditions leading to their severe disease and or death. **So, this author is not saying that there is no disease process occurring in society.** However, the understanding of the provenance and nature of the disease is crucial for determining the right treatment of the disease; and there are thousands of legitimate scientists that dispute the self-serving narratives and treatments that the politicians and health authorities

---
[3] https://news.yahoo.com/next-global-depression-coming-optimism-104042721.html

have instituted. Thus, whatever the disease might be, the manipulation of the disease process to promote fear, subjugation, and debilitation of society that lead to disease, disharmony and unnecessary suffering and death are the ethical issues being focused on here. The manipulation of the disease process through lies about the origins and effects of the disease process, the intentional and unintentional errors leading to public hysteria and psychosis, inter-family and inter social group conflict, outright scams for profit, that have led to deaths that can be considered in the context of homicide and murder, etc. are the issues to be confronted. In order to develop positively as opposed to descending into chaos, mentally and physically diseased servile obedience to sociopathic and psychopathic rulers, the society needs to face its pathologies so as to resolve them by growing in ethical and spiritual strength.

The ethical problems, surrounding the disease process, referred to as "coronavirus" or "covid 19", stem from the emerging evidence of apparent man-made creation or manipulation of existing viruses or some other agents (the virus has not been fully demonstrated) that led to the existence of the disease process referred to as "coronavirus" or "covid 19". Furthermore, the creation or manipulations of viruses could have been done specifically for the use of the disease process referred to as "coronavirus" or "covid 19" to establish totalitarian controls on the population. Other ethical issues include the way that the disease process has been used to instill fear in the population and justify the use of controversial ***experimental chemical therapies surreptitiously called vaccines***, supposedly to stem the disease. So, in short, there is apparently a disease process affecting a fraction, not all of the population. However, as of this writing, a particular virus has not been isolated and proven to be the sole cause of that disease process even though the messages to the public say it is a fact. Thus, the virus cause is only a hypothesis since a "virus" that causes the disease referred to as coronavirus or covid 19 has, up to now, not been isolated. Therefore, calling the disease process, whatever it may be, a "virus" is problematic since it characterizes the disease, and its possible treatments, in a way that can be manipulated.

Therefore, while the disease itself is real the falsehoods and schemes by medical officials, social media and politicians, and the use of it for the manipulation of society, through fear about it, are the frauds that are hurting, not helping the population. The deconstruction of these frauds, through Maatian ethical reflections and analysis, is a major part of this Volume 2 of MAAT VS FASCISM AND THE POLICE STATE.

An example, among many, of the frauds around the disease process, referred to as "coronavirus" or "covid 19", is that it should not be named since a definitive cause, be it a virus or something else, has not yet been proven. Another example, of the frauds around the disease process, referred to as "coronavirus" or "covid 19", is that contrary to the constant official announcements, it is not a disease that affects the entire population since not all members of the population are susceptible to it. These among other frauds will be discussed in this volume with the ideal of establishing an ethical basis for confronting the health, social, economic, and political challenges facing humanity.

Economic Malfeasance and Political Corruption in the Year 2020

In the year 2020, society, as a whole, continued imploding regarding the disease, general stress, and social discourse. The USA population also recorded a reduction in life expectancy, but the cause was not "coronavirus" or "covid 19". It was due to the deteriorating status of overall physical and emotional health and diminishing longevity of the population due to the toxicity of the culture including the economy, politics, social and family relationships, standard American diet (processed food and meat eating), air quality, health care, and overall diminishing quality of life, and diminishing feelings of well-being and happiness. The lockdowns also had a contributing general negative contributing effect.

IMF heightens warnings on corporate debt following central bank cuts[4]

The new round of zero interest rate policy and perpetual bailouts continued inflating economic bubbles that will inevitably contribute to global debt and impending global economic collapse, yet it is being done to evade an

---

[4] https://www.reuters.com/article/us-imf-worldbank-gfsr-idUSKBN1WV1N5

economic collapse caused by government and bank malfeasance and prolong the time of elite power and capacity to rapaciously take from the general economy to enrich a minority power elite and their employees. The term "Power Elite" refers to the richest minority of most powerful persons who control the commanding heights of the world economies in each country and globally including the transnational corporations. They leverage their power and control to coordinate actions that usurp the wealth of the world population, arrogate it for themselves and use that power to exert control and impose policies that diminish the wealth, power, and sovereignty of the masses while further enhancing their power and wealth to exert further control and exploitation of the masses of humanity. The term "power elite" maybe, for this study, equated with the terms "global elite" or "global power elite".

> In his 1956 book *The power elite*, sociologist C Wright Mills states that together with the military and political establishment, leaders of the biggest corporations form a "power elite" that is in control of the U.S.[5]

WHO ARE THE POWER ELITES?

> "There are invisible rulers who control the destinies of millions. It is not generally realized to what extent the words and actions of our most influential public men are dictated by shrewd persons operating behind the scenes."
> — Edward L. Bernays, Propaganda

The power elites are a minuscule segment of the world population that are so rich that they do not fly on commercial airlines, even in first class. They do not live with any classes (upper-middle, middle, or lower). They do not go to supermarkets or drive themselves anywhere. They have servants to do everything for them and they grow up in special prep schools that teach them that they are the master race that is entitled to rule over everyone else. They are taught, in school and at home, by having servants to boss around and make degrade themselves and grovel for pittances of reward in the form of subsistence currency, that everyone else, outside of their lives is insignificant fodder that they can manipulate or sacrifice to their greed and power designs. In other words, this is a culture and indoctrination/socialization scheme that fosters sociopathy in those who may be borderline sociopaths or acceptance of sociopathic values in those

---

[5] Doob, Christopher (2013). *Social Inequality and Social Stratification* (1st ed.). Boston: Pearson. p. 143.

who are so degraded by greed and lack of socialization with compassion and caring as to support the sociopaths in an effort to be in their "good graces". Yet, the true power elite does not have good graces, but only expedient utilitarian usages for those they can manipulate to their will; when that utility of the human fodder, their servants, is finished and has no further value, the human fodder is discarded. In the power elite paradigm, the "servants" are not just their butlers, maids, cooks, groundskeepers, drivers, etc. Their servants are whole populations the world over, from whom they extract wealth and manipulate into believing, feeling, and acting in accordance with their designs. In other words, they see the world population as their slaves, which they have the right to do with as they please, up to and including execution.[6] This power elite has the power to manipulate economies so that politicians who do not follow their policies would be forced to react, even by reluctantly going to war against other governments. They can engage in movements of money that destroy economies like that of the country Venezuela. They can financially support certain political leaders who will do their will or engage in a propaganda blitz that would destroy someone politically or even get someone, who does not follow their dictates, assassinated. When the fiction of the power elite paradigm is sufficiently understood and when there is sufficient pain in the populace to stimulate resistance, the power elites respond by introducing totalitarian police state tactics and codify those into the legal system. This is the state the USA and Western countries have reached. [7]

For the purposes of this study, to our primary name reference, **"power elite"**, we may include the definitions by psychiatrist Peter Breggin: **"Global Predators"**[8], by psychology professor, Jerry Kroth: **"The Parasitic Elite,"**[9] and Dr. Vernon Coleman: **"Evil Elite"**[10]. Another term that has been used is "globalist". The term "elite" refers to their social status, having elevated themselves above the rest of the population in terms of legal immunity, financial wealth and political power. The term "elite," as used here, does not refer to their ethics, or altruistic ideals; quite the opposite. They are elite in terms of high criminality, high sociopathy, high capacity to affect whole populations for their own designs and not for the good of humanity. From the Ancient Egyptian MAAT (truth in thought, speech, and action) wisdom perspective, they may be defined as: **"sneaky enemy"** and

---

[6] https://www.youtube.com/watch?v=PGwb3YQBW5k&t=604s
https://www.youtube.com/watch?v=o4WVPJWxAz8
[7] https://youtu.be/jPVzfuW72_M
[8] https://breggin.com/covid-19-and-the-global-predators-we-are-the-prey-latest-breggin-book/
[9] https://youtu.be/gOkaQPmftXg
[10] https://wisebird.com/

"**misleader**". This is essentially what would be considered in present-day terms as "**con artist**", an "**adversary**", a "**foe**", an "**antagonist**", a "**nemesis**". This type of personality is someone who means you harm but not necessarily openly but rather with subterfuge, one who uses trickery, deception, machination, duplicity, and schemes when possible and when that fails then manipulate people into conflict or employ the levers of government power to directly apply violence on the population through police and or military actions. The following translation of the Ancient Egyptian wisdom text of Amenemopet illustrates the Ancient Egyptian viewpoint about this type of personality.[11]

Teachings of Amenemopet Chapter 3

Verse 10.
10.1. im-an ari   nehbu   tjetje   ra ma pa   teha   ra betjenu cheft
10.2. do not   yoking   gossiping (mouth) behold that   argument (mouth) sneaky enemy
10.3. Desist from, abstain, cease, renounce joining with and gossiping with and watch out, definitely not getting into verbal arguments with the sneaky enemy, the heated person.

Verse 15.
15.1. pa   shemm   {cheft}   im   unut   tu-f
15.2. that   heated   (enemy)   in   hour   to-he
15.3. That heated person (who is the enemy) when they are in their time of heat...

Verse 16.
16.1. tuoaha   tu - khat   f   chaa   setenem {her} {mdj} f
16.2. reject   to-thee heart his abandon   misleading(person)(tie) he
16.3. ...you should reject them by turning your mind away from their mind and emotions. You should abandon them because they are misleading personalities...

---

[11] Translation by Dr. Muata Ashby ©2019

HOW THE POWER ELITE EXERCISE THEIR POWER

The power elites have two primary arms of power through which they exert their power from behind the scenes. The power elites operate to exercise control over the population through philosophical and social institutions such as think tanks and advisory councils such as the Council on Foreign Relations, the Bilderberg Group and World Economic Forum which directly control the centers of political power (presidents, prime ministers, etc.); those think tanks and advisory councils directly control transnational and national industries and extend their influence through universities and congressional lobbying groups. All of the aforesaid relates to the intellectual arm. The other arm of power operates through the worldwide network of international interconnected central banks that control whole economies and coordinate economic booms and busts.[12] The banking system controls who gets the wealth of the society and prevents the masses from becoming wealthy while redirecting the wealth to the minority power elite and their institutions of control. This means, among other things, that the power elite banks control which corporations get financing and thus which industries will be allowed to function. Therefore, if the preference is for fossil fuels instead of renewables, the fossil fuel based companies will get the most financing. Similarly, if the power elite preference is for polluting industries that may pollute the environment, even to the extent of or perhaps because of the deleterious effects on the male sperm count (for population reduction purposes), then the elites in control will impose those polluting industries on the world.[13] The preference of power elites, at the beginning of the 20th century, was for allopathic medical systems based on drugs instead of holistic health. That is how the current drug-based, germ theory based medical system came into being as other health systems, such as chiropractic and homeopathy, were suppressed by withdrawing financing from them and instituting a negative propaganda campaign against them ever since, thereby convincing the society that allopathic health systems are scientific and drug based science is the only real health system while all others are dangerous quacks. Additionally, they convinced the society that allopathic trained doctors are the only "true scientists" and other health modalities are not scientific. So too, the media companies that are desired by the power elite will get the financing and if they want to continue to get the financing they will not contradict the narratives of the power elite financed "opinion leaders", in other words, control and suppression of

---

[12] https://prn.fm/progressive-commentary-hour-05-19-21/
[13] https://www.wtsp.com/article/news/health/male-fertility-rate-sperm-count-falling/67-9f65ab4c-5e55-46d3-8aea-1843a227d848#:~:text=Brink%20of%20a%20fertility%20crisis,longer%20produce%20sperm%20by%202045.

information (censorship and propaganda). By financially supporting certain news companies and "leaders" the power elites foster belief systems (opinions) and through dependencies forced on news reporters and media companies, they oblige a dependency of journalists and news companies on politicians for news which compromises their ability to discover and pass on the truth to the population. Thereby the policies of the power elites, and the subjects of discussion, are controlled and disseminated to the population via the politicians and the news media.

> "But being dependent, every day of the year and for year after year, upon certain politicians for news, the newspaper reporters are obliged to work in harmony with their news sources."

> "No serious sociologist any longer believes that the voice of the people expresses any divine or specially wise and lofty idea. The voice of the people expresses the mind of the people, and that mind is made up for it by the group leaders in whom it believes and by those persons who understand the manipulation of public opinion. It is composed of inherited prejudices and symbols and cliches and verbal formulas supplied to them by the leaders."

>   — Edward L. Bernays, Propaganda

THE POWER ELITE PLAN FOR ECONOMIC DEVASTATION, SOCIAL DESTRUCTION AND REMAKING

The 2019 continuing banking malfeasance crisis signaled the impending collapse of the economic system as a whole. However, by January of 2020, it became clear that there was a supposed new virus that was appearing in the world. The symptoms and deaths attributed to the new virus, named "Sars Covid-19", touted as being related to a previous supposed (never proven) sars virus, were conflated with symptoms and deaths from other diseases such as the flu, pneumonia, and other causes of death to create a panic by causing people to believe that all the deaths were from that "new virus".

This manufactured scare was declared a pandemic. Then, governments, the world over, in a coordinated fashion, adopted similar responses, all of which had the effect, not of helping the health issue but instead they exacerbated it and that acted as a cover for governments to imposed totalitarian lockdowns later to be followed news castersby calls for a "vaccine" that could "save lives" and allow everyone to go back to "normal life." The lockdowns included suppressing social gatherings, dissent, and the questioning of the new policies, closing businesses and causing millions to panic and millions forced into bankruptcies. Those bankruptcies, as occurred in the financial crisis of 2008, allowed the rich, the corporations, and the banks to further profit by taking over bankrupt businesses and foreclosing on real estate properties, and by the purchase of business assets at pennies on the dollar. They also allowed industries to consolidate and become bigger while impoverishing the previous business owners and the employees of the companies they assimilated. The manufactured scare and subsequent response to the so-called "pandemic" in the form of lockdowns also gave cover to governments and banks so they could blame the pandemic on the failing economy and the need to "counterfeit" (create currency out of thin air) currency to sustain unemployed people, while in reality giving most of the currency to banks and big corporations. Thus, **in the year 2020,** there was a new excuse for the need to apply the failed strategy of lowering banking interest rates (which hurts savers) and create more currency, which helps those corporations that receive it while devaluing the rest of the currency (which causes inflation) that is already in existence, thereby stealing wealth from the general population, through inflation as the currency becomes worth less and less each time this is done.

Then, **in the year 2020**, began the greatest single-year injection of reserve currency than at any time in USA history, which would signal the accelerating destruction of the buying power of the US dollar and the increase in the price of gold and silver that occurs in an economic downfall. However, in this and other crises, most of the newly created currency went to the worldwide rich, the banks and the big corporations and not to those in most dire need or the middle class, the locked-down businesses, or the poor. This policy of 2020 was in harmony with the actions by president Obama in 2008-2009 when he bailed out all the banks and did nothing to stop millions of ordinary homeowners who were foreclosed on by those same banks that were bailed out; so, from that time on, the policy of everything for corporations and nothing for ordinary people (neo-liberalism) was on full display. In this context, Obama was the culmination, at that time, of the Corporatist presidency wherein the congress and presidency openly, unapologetically and without pretense, acted on behalf of corporations at the expense of the population.

Thus, by design, in the year 2020, the rich used the opportunity of a supposed medical crisis and the supposed need for lockdowns, to get richer[14] as the poor got poorer and yet the poor and middle classes continued to go along with the dictates of the authority figures and continued supporting and sometimes even defending them with blind allegiance. This may be considered an effect of almost a year of fear-mongering, media propaganda in support of the fear-mongering, and imposed dependency on the state (forcing business closures and lockdowns and giving limited handouts of cash called "stimulus payments").

Under such conditions, of the imposed social order, coupled with constant media propagandizing, supporting the fear-mongering, the psychological state of the society may be considered in the context of Stockholm syndrome. The populations in the countries that have experienced the propaganda and lockdowns have experienced a kind of hostage situation imposed by their governments similar to "Stockholm Syndrome". In Stockholm syndrome the effects of indoctrination, torture, and stress on a captive victim, causes them to lose personal sovereignty and capacity for clear thought and reflection sufficient for making decisions that can provide for personal wellbeing. The syndrome causes them to believe in and accept the position, legitimacy, and goodness of the captor/torturer/murderer and even defend the captor/torturer, even after being freed from captivity. This particular issue has been cited in reference to people who have been kidnapped, abducted, or abused by spouses or family members, who support and defend the abusers and later go back to them and receive more abuse, but this syndrome also applies to populations that have been abused and conditioned by political captors and their technical assistants, the bureaucracy that does the actual management of society on their behalf and on their directions with orders that are meant to instill fear, perpetrate propaganda, increase control, loss of rights and exploit the population while convincing people they, the power elite, have the best interests, of the people, at heart. An example of this is the now president Joe Biden who, as a senator, was the author of a crime bill that brought perhaps the largest increase in incarceration in the history of the country, including for non-violent crimes; additionally, he authored the "patriot act" that took human rights away and ushered in a surveillance police state; he also authored a bill supporting the financial sector that led to the 2008 crash of the economy and continuing collapse of the economy. He is also responsible for the incapacity of students to get out from under predatory student loans.

---

[14] **HOW BILLIONAIRES SAW THEIR NET WORTH INCREASE BY HALF A TRILLION DOLLARS DURING THE PANDEMIC**
Hiatt Woods Oct 30, 2020, 5:30 PM- https://www.businessinsider.com/billionaires-net-worth-increases-coronavirus-pandemic-2020-7?op=1

Together with Barak Obama, Biden helped orchestrate the destruction of the country, Libya, with lies about the country and its leaders and helped start other wars with him. Yet, in the year 2020, he (Biden) was accepted as a legitimate and even benevolent leader. Other authority figures such as Ronald Reagan, Bill Clinton, and Barak Obama, who could make people feel good with their words and manners, were not criticized or prosecuted for their moral and or legal transgressions and war crimes and are still praised by their followers, many years after being out of office. Thus, the "war on terror" which was started as a response to the attacks of 9/11/01, which was the latest in the history of false flag events used as excuses for political distraction, drumming up patriotic support for aggression against other countries and curtailing civil right, morphed into the new war on covid. Which is apparently a conflict born of a manmade weapon of mass destruction now used as an excuse for fomenting aggression between citizens within the country, fear, curtailing more civil rights, and impoverishing the population.

When a person's sense of autonomy and sovereignty are surpassed by a desire for comfort, convenience, security, and or apathy, then as Aldus Huxley[15] would see it, people willingly give up their freedom in exchange for "feeling good"; the feeling good is like a medication that dulls the sense capacity to perceive what is detrimental in the long run so there is continual reliance on "feel-good" substitutes such as TV shows, "feel-good" medications, "feel-good" words from friends or politicians, "feel-good" clicks from social media, etc. When the "feel-good" inputs are not received then they attack the source they identify as the reason they cannot experience the perceived mental relief, confused with peace, that comes from self-delusion, regardless of if it is coming from a source of honesty or not. Delusion is a mental illness that can lead people to commit heinous acts of violence and self-destruction.[16] So at this point, "feeling-good" has become more important than living by the truth and this self-deluding movement in the personality leads to enslavement by the same desired comforts and conveniences. The lure of the same desired comforts and conveniences is used by unethical, immoral, amoral, and or criminal con-artist corporate and political leaders who promise, like common street drug pushers, to continue supplying the means for more self-delusion, but neglect to let on that this is a process of disempowerment and political as well as economic impoverishment. People do not, or are unable to, look at these

---

[15] **BRAVE NEW WORLD 1932**
[16] Prof. Jerry Kroth Propaganda and Manipulation: How mass media engineers and distorts our perceptions   https://youtu.be/Pfo5gPG72KM

personalities (the unethical, immoral, amoral, and or criminal con-artist corporate and political leaders) critically; otherwise, those demonstrably toxic personalities would not be accepted for any kind of leadership position.

The capacity for critical thinking and autonomous decision-making has been compromised and atrophied, due to the social traumas and personal, mental, physical, and emotional damage caused by decades of living lives of self-delusion, not living by truth (MAAT). Individuals within such a society of untruth live lives of stunted maturity and are therefore infantilized and relegated to seeking approval and permission from authority (parent) figures in order to feel as if they were thinking and acting out of their own volition. In the present context, people who are dominated, propagandized and surveilled, censored, and whose choices in government or economics are limited by the power elite cannot, by definition, have individual volition as their mental capacity and choices are all corrupted and therefore compromised from the beginning. Therefore, the idea of personal choice or freedom is illusory in the context of domination by an overarching power elite paradigm. This idea of being a pawn in the designs of a power elite personality should be repugnant to a self-respecting person; yet the world population accepts the situation and deludes itself as to its rights and choice capacities, ceding the power of physical and mental control to power elites that are themselves compromised by their delusions of power that lead to reckless disregard for the safety and wellbeing of humanity, animals and the environment as well as their own health and wellbeing.

The populations of societies worldwide, composed of personalities with reduced cognitive and ethical capacity, allows the worst elements of society (kakistocracy), not only common criminals, but criminal sociopaths, to lead the society while partaking in self-defeating debilitating lifestyles. Those self-defeating debilitating lifestyles include legal and illegal drug abuse, unhealthy stressful lifestyles, pleasure-seeking, and engaging in empty, instead of engaging in uplifting and empowering, spiritual practices that enrich the spirit and provide spiritual strength, along with ethical and moral fortitude. People have degraded to and are encouraged by religious and political demagogues and rapacious corporate leaders, supported by compromised media personalities and celebrities to engage in actions that instead impoverish body and spirit while empowering and enriching sociopaths and compromised greedy individuals whose morality has been subsumed under the ocean of avaricious thoughts and desires.

THE YEAR 2020 REVEALED FASCISM AND THE POLICE STATE IN ASCENDANCY...

The year 2020 revealed some important aspects of human society that are important considerations related to *Maat vs. Fascism and the Police State*. Firstly, it revealed that the phenomenon of firing workers and not replacing or rehiring them, after a supposed economic recession or in this case, an economic crash, especially if they are in the manufacturing sector, occurred again, in the year 2020, as in 2008-09; this was a reapplication of the excuse to accelerate the getting rid of workers in favor of automation and technological substitutes such as artificial intelligence, as well as lower-paid workers. Thus, this is not only a reaction to economic downturns in a capitalist system of economics but a specific tactic, using a crisis as an excuse, to replace workers with outsourcing and automation to reduce costs. So workers are treated increasingly as disposable commodities.

The year 2020 revealed the extent to which human beings are very susceptible to directives by authority figures. Initially, most people readily complied with directives to wear facemasks and close down their businesses, and stay home to supposedly cope with a supposed "pandemic". But when information started to come out pointing to the fact that the virus was not as deadly as first thought and that mask-wearing, social-distancing and lockdowns do more harm than good, people continued to obey the authority figures and the media that kept touting their efficacy and the need for the continued imposition of the lockdowns on society.

The year 2020 revealed how people, after suffering the blow of the major 2008 financial crisis and decades of economic stagnation and real wages not rising, education systems becoming costly and tending towards indoctrination for supporting government and corporations instead of ethics and the humanities, has led to a younger generation that is susceptible to social media, instead of being influenced by humanities-based classical wisdom, for their feelings of self-worth and moral, ethical conscience. They are also susceptible, by not having a proper guide of moral and ethical conscience, to the social media identity politics, and to the demagoguery of the neoliberal and or neoconservative ideologies, which do not have the good of anyone, except their proponents and adherents, the power elite and transnational corporations, at heart.

The year 2020 revealed unprecedented and far-reaching as well as naked, open censorship in the general mainstream media and particularly from social media companies. This issue has become so dire that people on social media channels constantly announce they are self-censoring so as not to be removed from the platforms. Also, social media companies are removing, shadow banning, or relegating books and other materials deemed by them as contradictory to the prevailing government or authority figure narratives, to the back of search engine results.[17]

The year 2020 revealed how the state (in collusion with the central bank) has stolen wealth from the population, through reserve banking and inflation as well as through unlawful income taxation.[18] Another source of theft is the police system itself under a program called "Civil Asset Forfeiture", whereby property is simply taken from citizens, by police, without any probable cause or law being proven as having being violated by them; the property is simply confiscated under the pretext of suspicion by a law enforcement officer.[19]

The year 2020 revealed how quickly and easily and how the vast quantity of the population were willing to believe the statements of pathological lying politicians and criminal corporations by blindly submitting themselves to the unscientific, contradictory, and discredited decrees, not laws, imposed by presidents, prime ministers, governors, etc. The same year revealed how easily most of the population would accept the term, "lockdown", to be applied to themselves, which was previously associated with prisons that lockdown inmates. Thereby the fear traumatized, gullible, naïve and simple-minded as well as the stupid and ignorant smart people that also go along, accepted the moniker of an inmate in the mandated closed air prison of their homes, hoping things would somehow go back to "normal" if they obey the "authorities". The same year revealed how quickly and easily most people accepted the irrational dictates such as mask wearing. Mask wearing became normalized even though masks cannot protect from viruses. Thus, the dangerous and useless but mandated gesture (wearing masks) became a means to block human communication and have a focus point (in your face), a constant reminder of irrational fear and symbols of obedience to and control by the power elite. From the

---

[17] https://www.corbettreport.com/episode-384-the-library-of-alexandria-is-on-fire/
[18] https://archive.org/details/freedom_to_fascism
https://www.youtube.com/watch?v=ZKeaw7HPG04
[19] https://www.briansilber.com/police-have-taken-68-billion-in-20-years-without-due-process-thanks-to-civil-asset-forfeiture-report-reveals/
https://ammo.com/articles/civil-asset-forfeiture-policing-for-profit

perspective of the mask wearer, they have been convinced to be fearful of contracting "corona virus" or spreading it, asymptomatically, to a loved one; beliefs that are based on lies. From the perspective of the power elites, the mask wearing is a form of obedience training, not unlike dog training or circus animal training. In fact, obedience to all of the irrational, contradictory and outrageous impositions and police brutalities for not being obedient are obedience training, leading to further acceptance of more power elite impositions. The same symbols of oppression, fear and delusion, were turned, by the duped wearers, into colorful and artistic designer fashion statements muzzling their freedom of expression and adorning their own acquiescence and obedience to oppression and delusion. The lockdowns have been proven to be unscientific, and to not prevent[20] disease. In some cases the lockdowns promote more infection, disease, despair, stress, domestic abuse, and suicides, while many people continue waiting in fear for an authority figure to say it is ok to come out from hiding. In the meantime, the lockdowns caused more infections since it was discovered that most infections occur in the household, indoors and not outside. This is an example of how the failed strategy of lockdowns, preventing people from getting fresh air and sunlight, causes more harm. Yet the policy continues to be pushed by politicians and the media as of this writing.

CDC study says tons of people catch COVID-19 in the one place that's supposed to be safe[21]
October 31st, 2020

- The CDC published a new coronavirus study that looked at the infection rate inside the household.
- Researchers found that 102 out of 191 people who came in contact with a sick person contracted COVID-19, with transmission likely occurring inside the home.
- 75% of the secondary household infections happened within 5 days, and researchers observed "substantial transmission" whether the first patient was a child or an adult.

A rational person may think of the imposition of social practices that are proven incorrect as being wrong actions or as mistakes. However, when we consider that those who are benefitting **from**

---

[20] https://youtu.be/Ay12R0e_7WM
[21] https://bgr.com/2020/10/31/coronavirus-transmission-at-home-cdc-study/

the supposed "wrong" policies, such as facemask wearing, lockdowns, and social distancing, are the same ones (tech companies, big pharmaceutical companies, the CDC, and power elite individuals such as Bill Gates and Anthony Fauci) directing it and when we also consider that the supposedly scientific-minded and scientifically trained medical professionals, who should be the ones rejecting the "wrong" policies are not acting according to science[22] and are not rejecting the "wrong" policies and are even supporting them, we may justifiably suspect that they are willingly or ignorantly following the direction of someone who has control over them, who wants those policies to be imposed for their purposes, which do not include promoting health. From this, we may also conclude that the policy that seems "wrong" or a "mistake" to a regular non-power elite person is indeed correct from the power elite perspective. For a person who is a member of the power elite, who is sociopathic and or overcome by the desire for power and wealth, the injurious policies are a means to the end of achieving the goals they are working for, instilling fear, impoverishment, domination, and exploitation. The control over the medical profession and demonstration of its corruption was attested to by prominent members of the medical-industrial complex including a professor of Medicine at Harvard University and former Editor-in-Chief of the New England Medical Journal.[23]

Harvard Professor Says Prescription Drugs Are Killing Population

A Harvard Professor has claimed that prescription drugs are not only ineffective at treating most illnesses but are actually killing the population.

========

The End of Evidence-Based Medicine and The Rise of Medical Propaganda

---

[22] VIRUS MANIA: CORONA/COVID-19, MEASLES, SWINE FLU, CERVICAL CANCER, AVIAN FLU, SARS, BSE, HEPATITIS C, AIDS, POLIO, SPANISH FLU. HOW THE MEDICAL ... MAKING BILLION-DOLLAR PROFITS AT OUR EXPENSE PAPERBACK – JANUARY 28, 2021
[23] https://drfarrah.online/end-evidence-based-medicine-rise-medical-propaganda/
https://drjasonfung.medium.com/the-corruption-of-evidence-based-medicine-killing-for-profit-41f2812b8704

LIES, FACEMASKS, SOCIAL DISTANCING, AND LOCKDOWNS

Masks Are Neither Effective Nor Safe: A Summary Of The Science[24]

The year 2020 revealed the extent to which the authority figures in government and in the supposed government agencies responsible for health were willing to lie about the level of danger of the virus, and the need to use facemasks, social distancing, and lockdowns even as evidence accumulated, by summer 2020, that their mandates were not based on science but rather on arbitrary, unscientific falsehoods told by politicians and supposed health professionals along with the media. Facemasks and social distancing and "lockdowns" have been found to be ineffective for controlling the virus spread, in the general population, and are rather more injurious than the virus. In fact, facemasks, and therefore, mask mandates cause infection and debilitate the immune system causing disease rates to climb instead of going down.[25]

Dr. Fauci Made the Coronavirus Pandemic Worse by Lying About Masks[26] 6/16/2020

> Anthony Fauci has been hailed as a hero during the coronavirus pandemic, delivering thoughtful health advice… Simply put, Fauci lied about whether masks were helpful in slowing the spread of the virus.

The political and medical authorities claim to be "following the science" in dealing with covid 19 disease. If they are following the science why did then NOT follow the findings of the New England Journal of Medicine about mask wearing:

---

[24] Masks Are Neither Effective Nor Safe: A Summary Of The Science
https://www.technocracy.news/masks-are-neither-effective-nor-safe-a-summary-of-the-science/
NEW DANISH STUDY FINDS MASKS DON'T PROTECT WEARERS FROM COVID INFECTION
https://fee.org/articles/new-danish-study-finds-masks-don-t-protect-wearers-from-covid-infection/
[25] ttps://www.drbvip.com/
[26] https://www.msn.com/en-us/news/us/dr-fauci-made-the-coronavirus-pandemic-worse-by-lying-about-masks/ar-BB15zyW3

> New England Journal of Medicine stated on May 21, 2020 that "We know that wearing a mask outside health care facilities offers little, if any, protection from infection."[27]

Instead of following the scientific findings the political and medical authorities instead, on June 3, 2020: the authors of this article were required to contradict themselves and agree with the political policy and not their scientific findings:

> "We strongly support the calls of public health agencies for all people to wear masks when circumstances compel them to be within 6 ft of others for sustained periods."

> **Editor's Note:** This article was published on April 1, 2020, at NEJM.org. In a letter to the editor on June 3, 2020, the authors of this article state "We strongly support the calls of public health agencies for all people to wear masks when circumstances compel them to be within 6 ft of others for sustained periods."

Conclusion: The "public health agencies" are *NOT* "following the science." They are following a propaganda agenda in coordination with ulterior motives and supporting mask wearing which maintains personal and constant fear in the population.

The Initial Fauci Lie about Mask Wearing was not a lie. The lie was the subsequent retraction from the initial statement made by Mr. Fauci.

Many people, in alternative media, have pointed out that Anthony Fauci lied about mask wearing when he and the surgeon general were initially saying that masks do not work. This logic presupposes that masks actually do work for preventing viral infections. When Fauci and the supposed health authorities revered their previous statements and then were in favor of wearing masks that was taken as the admittance of the initial lie.

However, when the evidences about mask wearing are examined, it turns out that in the beginning Fauci was actually telling the truth. Tests on masks in previous years and also throughout the year 2020 proved that masks do not prevent infections from viruses, they are too small and pass through the masks. So the retraction from the earlier statement that masks do not work, that was the start of the lying about mask wearing as a protection from corona virus. That lie facilitated the ever-present reminder in everyone's

---

[27] https://www.nejm.org/doi/full/10.1056/NEJMp2006372

immediate awareness (on their face) of a supposed deadly pathogen that requires fear of the environment and fear of other people as possible carriers. The understanding that the "corona virus" is no more deadly (in fact less deadly) than the annual FLU means that the gran deception that people have fallen for and the grand deceivers perpetrating and perpetuating the deception, are examples of a society wherein reality and truth have become illusory spectacles themselves; thus the society cannot function in a reality-based context and will continue to be victimized by delusions, be they about illusory viruses or illusory weapons of mass destruction.

Fauci Admits He's Been Lying to Us About Herd Immunity In Order to Manipulate Us[28]| Dec 28, 2020

===========

Dr. Peter Mcullough:
"We are at 80% herd immunity right now without the vaccine effect… the vaccine is going to have 1% public health impact, that's what the data says, its not going to save us; we are already 80% herd immune." (March 10, 2021)[29]

Natural Herd Immunity is an issue denied by the health officials and the mainstream media. Studies now show that people who may have been infected with and suffered symptoms or perhaps even did not suffer symptoms of the disease referred to as "corona virus" or "covid 19" have developed lasting natural immunity as evidenced by the finding of antibodies even a year later. The denial of these findings, by the health authorities and the mainstream news media points to an agenda of promoting the absence of alternatives to receiving experimental vaccines that, up to this time, their level and duration of protection from infection has not been proven but their incapacity to protect from infections has been already demonstrated by the increasing numbers of "breakthrough cases" that have been detected. The CDC announced they will stop counting the

---

[28] https://redstate.com/brandon_morse/2020/12/28/fauci-admits-hes-been-lying-to-us-about-herd-immunity-in-order-to-manipulate-us-n300795
[29] https://youtu.be/lL6U31QKOQc
https://youtu.be/Jkwn5I8tLmE

"breakthrough cases";[30] this action is being taken so as not to interfere with the vaccine uptake, in other words, not to cause people to question the efficacy of the experimental chemical gene therapies referred to as "vaccines."

---

https://www.cdc.gov/vaccines/covid-19/health-departments/breakthrough-cases.html

May 1, 2021, CDC transitioned from monitoring all reported vaccine breakthrough...

Defining a vaccine breakthrough infection

For the purpose of this surveillance, a vaccine breakthrough infection is defined as the detection of SARS-CoV-2 RNA or antigen in a respiratory specimen collected from a person ≥14 days after they have completed all recommended doses of a U.S. Food and Drug Administration (FDA)-authorized COVID-19 vaccine.

Identifying and investigating hospitalized or fatal vaccine breakthrough cases

As of **May 1, 2021, CDC transitioned from monitoring all reported vaccine breakthrough cases to focus on identifying and investigating only hospitalized or fatal cases due to any cause.** This shift will help maximize the quality of the data collected on cases of greatest clinical and public health importance.

---

https://www.cdc.gov/mmwr/volumes/70/wr/mm7021e3.htm

COVID-19 Vaccine Breakthrough Infections Reported to CDC — United States, January 1–April 30, 2021
Early Release / May 25, 2021 / 70

A total of 10,262 SARS-CoV-2 vaccine breakthrough infections had been reported from 46 U.S. states and territories as of April 30, 2021.

- **6,446** (63%) occurred in females
- median patient age was 58 years (interquartile range = 40–74 years)
- **2,725** (27%) vaccine breakthrough infections were asymptomatic
- **995** (10%) patients were known to be hospitalized
- **160** (2%) patients died.

---

[30] **C.D.C. Will Not Investigate Mild Infections in Vaccinated Americans**
At least 10,000 vaccinated people were infected with the coronavirus through the end of April. Now the agency has stopped pursuing the mildest cases.
https://www.nytimes.com/2021/05/25/health/cdc-coronavirus-infections-vaccine.html
CDC has stopped counting every 'breakthrough' Covid infection in fully vaccinated people: Experts warn agency's new method of only collecting data on patients who are hospitalized or die could miss patterns in who gets sick after their shots
https://www.dailymail.co.uk/health/article-9566619/CDC-stopped-counting-breakthrough-Covid-infection-fully-vaccinated-people.html

https://www.theepochtimes.com/face-mask-mandates-seem-to-make-ccp-virus-infection-rates-climb-says-study_3629627.html?utm_source=morningbriefnoe&utm_medium=email&utm_campaign=mb-2020-12-23

US NEWS

Mask Mandates Seem to Make CCP Virus Infection Rates Climb, Study Says

Researchers examined cases covering a 229-day period running from May 1 through Dec. 15 and compared the days in which state governments had imposed mask mandates and the days when they hadn't.

In states with a mandate in effect, there were 9,605,256 confirmed COVID-19 cases, which works out to an average of 27 cases per 100,000 people per day.

When states didn't have a statewide order—including states that never had mandates, coupled with the period of time masking states didn't have the mandate in place—there were 5,781,716 cases, averaging 17 cases per 100,000 people per day.

In other words, protective-mask mandates have a poor track record so far in fighting the coronavirus. States with mandates in place produced an average of 10 more reported infections per 100,000 people per day than states without mandates.

The 15 states that went without a statewide mask mandate for the duration of the analysis were Alaska, Arizona, Florida, Georgia, Idaho, Iowa, Missouri, North Dakota, Nebraska, New Hampshire, Oklahoma, South Carolina, South Dakota, Tennessee, and Wyoming, ..

Face masks restrict the elimination of virus, recirculating the virus into the nasal/sinus and upper respiratory passages-

- "By wearing a mask, the exhaled viruses will not be able to escape and will concentrate in the nasal passages, enter the olfactory nerves and travel into the brain." Article by **Russell Blaylock M.D., published May 14, 2020 in Technocracy News & Trends.** Dr. Blaylock is a prominent retired neurosurgeon and author of health-related books. "We know that people who have the worst reactions to the coronavirus have the highest concentrations of the virus early on. And this leads to the deadly cytokine storm in a selected number." (Blaylock: Face Masks Pose Serious Risks To The Healthy; https://www.technocracy.news/blaylock-face-masks-pose-serious-risks-to-the-healthy/)
- This direct rebreathing of the virus back into the nasal passages can contribute to the migration of the virus to the brain. (1, 2) "Newer evidence suggests that in some cases the virus can enter the brain. In most instances it enters the brain by way of the olfactory nerves (smell nerves), which connect directly with the area of the brain dealing with recent memory and memory consolidation. By wearing a mask, the exhaled viruses will not be able to escape and will concentrate in the nasal passages, enter the olfactory nerves and travel into the brain."(3)

1. Baig AM et al. *Evidence of the COVID-19 virus targeting the CNS: Tissue distribution, host-virus interaction, and proposed neurotropic mechanisms.* ACS https://pubmed.ncbi.nlm.nih.gov/32187747/ ;.998.
2. Wu Y et al. *Nervous system involvement after infection with COVID-19 and other coronaviruses.* Brain Behavior, and Immunity.
3. Perlman S et al. *Spread of a neurotropic murine coronavirus into the CNS via the trigeminal and olfactory nerves.* Virology 1989;170:556-560.

Face Masks

https://bmjopen.bmj.com/content/bmjopen/5/4/e006577.full.pdf
https://www.ncbi.nlm.nih.gov/pmc/articles/PMC4420971/

"This study is the first RCT of cloth masks, and the results caution against the use of cloth masks. This is an important finding to inform occupational health and safety. Moisture retention, reuse of cloth masks and poor filtration may result **in increased risk of infection.**"

https://www.acpjournals.org/doi/10.7326/M20-1342

"In conclusion, both surgical and cotton masks seem to be ineffective in preventing the dissemination of SARS–CoV-2 from the coughs of patients with COVID-19 to the environment and external mask surface."

https://www.medrxiv.org/content/10.1101/2020.04.01.20049528v1?ijkey=5cc463fb85e2222477e813c7f859860174e11198&keytype2=tf_ipsecsha

"The evidence is not sufficiently strong to support widespread use of facemasks as a protective measure against COVID-19. However, there is enough evidence to support the use of facemasks for short periods of time by particularly vulnerable individuals when in transient higher risk situations."

---

https://www.technocracy.news/new-danish-study-face-masks-dont-protect-against-covid/

This Danish study proves what many medical professionals have stated all along: Face masks are useless against the spread of a virus. It's time to pop the Technocrat coup d'etat bubble once and for all. - TN Editor

A newly released study in the academic journal *Annals of Internal Medicine* casts more doubt on policies that force healthy individuals to wear face coverings in hopes of limiting the spread of COVID-19.

"Researchers in Denmark reported on Wednesday that surgical masks did not protect the wearers against infection with the coronavirus in a large randomized clinical trial," the *New York Times* reports. To conduct the study, which ran from early April to early June, scientists at the University of Copenhagen recruited more than 6,000 participants who had tested negative for COVID-19 immediately prior to the experiment.

Half the participants were given surgical masks and instructed to wear them outside the home; the other half were instructed to not wear a mask outside the home.

Roughly 4,860 participants finished the experiment, the *Times* reports. The results were not encouraging.

"The researchers had hoped that masks would cut the infection rate by half among wearers. Instead, 42 people in the mask group, or 1.8 percent, got infected, compared with 53 in the unmasked group, or 2.1 percent. The difference was not statistically significant," the *Times* reports.

> **https://swprs.org/face-masks-evidence/**
> Swiss Policy Research
>
> ### Studies on the effectiveness of face masks
>
> So far, most studies found little to **no evidence for the effectiveness of cloth face masks in the general population, neither as personal protective equipment nor as a source control.**
>
> 1. A May 2020 meta-study on pandemic influenza published by the **US CDC** found that **face masks had no effect, neither as personal protective equipment nor as a source control.** (Source)
>
> 2. A **Danish randomized controlled trial** with 6000 participants, published in the Annals of Internal Medicine in November 2020, **found no statistically significant effect of high-quality medical face masks against SARS-CoV-2 infection in a community setting.** (Source)
>
> 3. A July 2020 review by the **Oxford Centre for Evidence-Based Medicine** found that there is **no evidence for the effectiveness of cloth masks against virus infection or transmission.** (Source)
>
> 4. A May 2020 cross-country study by the **University of East Anglia** (preprint) found that **a mask requirement was of no benefit and could even increase the risk of infection.** (Source)
>
> 5. An April 2020 review by two US professors in respiratory and infectious disease from the **University of Illinois** concluded that **face masks have no effect in everyday life, neither as self-protection nor to protect third parties** (so-called source control). (Source)

https://wwwnc.cdc.gov/eid/article/26/5/19-0994_article
https://www.acpjournals.org/doi/10.7326/M20-6817
https://www.cebm.net/covid-19/masking-lack-of-evidence-with-politics/
https://www.medrxiv.org/content/10.1101/2020.05.01.20088260v1.full.pdf
https://www.cidrap.umn.edu/news-perspective/2020/04/commentary-masks-all-covid-19-not-based-sound-data

> **https://swprs.org/face-masks-evidence/**
> Swiss Policy Research
>
> ### Studies on the effectiveness of face masks
>
> 6. An article in the **New England Journal of Medicine** from **May 2020** came to the conclusion that **cloth face masks offer little to no protection in everyday life.** (Source)
>
> 7. An April 2020 **Cochrane review** (preprint) found that **face masks didn't reduce influenza-like illness (ILI) cases, neither in the general population nor in health care workers.** (Source)
>
> 8. An April 2020 review by the **Norwich School of Medicine** (preprint) found that "the evidence is not sufficiently strong to support widespread use of facemasks", but supports the use of masks by "particularly vulnerable individuals when in transient higher risk situations."
> https://www.medrxiv.org/content/10.1101/2020.04.01.20049528v1?ikey=5cc463fb85e2222477e813c7f859860174e11198&keytype2=tf_ipsecsha
>
> 9. A 2015 study in the British Medical Journal **BMJ Open** found that **cloth masks were penetrated by 97% of particles and may increase infection risk by retaining moisture or repeated use.**
> https://bmjopen.bmj.com/content/bmjopen/5/4/e006577.full.pdf
> https://www.ncbi.nlm.nih.gov/pmc/articles/PMC4420971
>
> 10. An August 2020 review by a **German professor** in virology, epidemiology and hygiene found that there is **no evidence for the effectiveness of cloth face masks and that the improper daily use of masks by the public may in fact lead to an increase in infections.** https://stillnessinthestorm.com/2020/10/german-neurologist-warns-against-wearing-facemasks-oxygen-deprivation-causes-permanent-neurological-damage/

https://www.nejm.org/doi/full/10.1056/NEJMp2006372
https://www.medrxiv.org/content/10.1101/2020.03.30.20047217v2

> **Face Masks**
>
> https://wwwnc.cdc.gov/eid/article/26/5/19-0994_article
>
> "**In this review, we did not find evidence to support a protective effect of personal protective measures or environmental measures in reducing influenza transmission.** Although these measures have mechanistic support based on our knowledge of how influenza is transmitted from person to person, randomized trials of hand hygiene and face masks have not demonstrated protection against laboratory-confirmed influenza..." and
>
> "**We did not find evidence that surgical-type face masks are effective in reducing laboratory-confirmed influenza transmission, either when worn by infected persons (source control) or by persons in the general community to reduce their susceptibility**"
>
> In conclusion, unless you are used to wearing a mask and the mask fits properly there is a tendency to constantly adjust the mask, touch your face, and scratch your nose not only making the mask irrelevant but increasing your risk. **After only a few minutes of wear, moisture develops inside the mask trapping natural respiratory pathogens from your nose and mouth causing potential reinfection and making the mask more permeable to outside pathogens. Unless the mask is properly vented, CO2 can build up which is very unhealthy causing headache, dizziness and respiratory distress.**
>
> This is a very concise summary of key points https://www.sott.net/article/434290-Russel-Blaylock-Face-masks-pose-serious-risks-to-the-healthy

Study Shows How Masks Are Harming Children

Analysis by Dr. Joseph Mercola[31]

---

[31] https://articles.mercola.com/sites/articles/archive/2021/02/27/effects-of-mask-mandates-and-school-closures.aspx?ui=152220df1deda081f73727bc10a8407027b248ba493a7ce71f4a1e73a6c1d882&sd=20200829&cid_source=dnl&cid_medium=email&cid_content=art2HL&cid=20210227_HL2&mid=DM816135&rid=1094715252

> https://www.researchsquare.com/article/rs-124394/v1
> **Corona children studies "Co-Ki": First results of a Germany-wide registry on mouth and nose covering (mask) in children**
>
> **Background:** Narratives about complaints in children and adolescents caused by wearing a mask are accumulating. There is, to date, no registry for side effects of masks.
> **Methods:** At the University of Witten/Herdecke an online registry has been set up where parents, doctors, pedagogues and others can enter their observations. On 20.10.2020, 363 doctors were asked to make entries and to make parents and teachers aware of the registry.
> **Results:** By 26.10.2020 the registry had been used by 20,353 people. In this publication we report the results from the parents, who entered **data on a total of 25,930 children. The average wearing time of the mask was 270 minutes per day. Impairments caused by wearing the mask were reported by 68% of the parents. These included irritability (60%), headache (53%), difficulty concentrating (50%), less happiness (49%), reluctance to go to school/kindergarten (44%), malaise (42%) impaired learning (38%) and drowsiness or fatigue (37%).**
> **Discussion:** This world's first registry for recording the effects of wearing masks in children is dedicated to a new research question. The frequency of the registry's use and the spectrum of symptoms registryed indicate the importance of the topic and call for representative surveys, randomized controlled trials with various masks and a renewed risk-benefit assessment for the vulnerable group of children: adults need to collectively reflect the circumstances under which they would be willing to take a residual risk upon themselves in favor of enabling children to have a higher quality of life without having to wear a mask.

So, while the evidence for mask-wearing shows either no benefit or no statistical difference between wearing a mask and not wearing a mask, in terms of protecting from the virus, but also shows real harms of prolonged universal mask-wearing by healthy individuals and children continues. The detriments (increased infection, re-inhaling the same air, getting less oxygen, psychological damage to adults and children, etc.) of prolonged wearing of masks by healthy individuals in the general population cause more harms than any discernable benefits. Additionally, it became known, by summer 2020, that asymptomatic carriers and children do not spread the disease so lockdowns, social distancing, school closures, and masks are not necessary in the first place.

More research showing that masks do not work:
Conclusion Regarding Masks: They Do Not Work by Dr. Sherri Tenpenny
https://vaxxter.com/coronavirus-pt-4-masks-dont-protect/
https://vaxxter.com/wp-content/uploads/2020/07/Masks-Final.pdf

Fallacy of Social-Distancing & Lockdowns

There is no science showing that social distancing is effective to prevent the spread of infection. Studies do show that asymptomatic persons do not spread disease.[32] Therefore, there is no scientific necessity or justification for lockdowns. So if anyone should socially distance themselves from others or participate in a quarantine it is those individuals who are sick. This is what people do in general, and have done for generations; if a person knows they are sick they stay home, which is natural and voluntary social distancing and self-quarantining[33], by the affected populations, until their disease passes.

Lockdowns on the general population do not work to prevent coronavirus disease.[34] Throughout history, lockdowns (which should really be called "quarantines" were never implemented on healthy populations until the present. Some scientists protested in the beginning and throughout the imposition of lockdowns, which were supposedly only to last 2 weeks to get coronavirus under control but actually have never been stopped. Yet, doctors and nurses went along with the lockdowns, and the policy was implemented nonetheless and continues to be carried out even now. Later, the WHO changed its guidance about lockdowns, and yet they continued to be implemented by governments around the world, even as they claim to be following the guidance from the WHO; such continued use of the discredited policy should be recognized as a red flag that the authorities continuing to impose the policies have an ulterior motive, other than promoting health, and that they are unfit for their leadership positions. These factors rightly cause many people to refer to medical tyrannical doctors, nurses, politicians and health officials as an unscientific "death cult".[35]

---

[32] https://www.bitchute.com/video/oUeNGpQVOHmA/
[33] https://wisebird.com/
[34] https://youtu.be/Ay12R0e_7WM
[35] https://brandnewtube.com/watch/dr-christiane-northrup-new-details-on-c-19-injections_gRTnpGJqPQg4Ndz.html

Social Distancing

https://amgreatness.com/2020/05/04/the-failed-experiment-of-social-distancing/

"social distancing" is untested pseudoscience particularly as it relates to halting the transmission of the SARS-CoV-2 virus. On its website, the CDC provides no links to any peer-reviewed social distancing studies that bolster its official guidance

https://www.americanthinker.com/articles/2020/05/social_distancing_is_snake_oil_not_science.html

"Very likely, you already instinctively know that the guidelines suggesting that it's somehow helpful to keep a six-foot space between healthy people, even outdoors, is not based on science, but just an arbitrary suggestion we've been conditioned to accept without evidence.

https://inside.upmc.com/shapiro-economy-roundtable/ (Dr Steven Shapiro) "What we cannot do, is extended social isolation. Humans are social beings, and we are already seeing the adverse mental health consequences of loneliness, and that is before the much greater effects of economic devastation take hold on the human condition."

https://rationalground.com/university-of-florida-researchers-find-no-asymptomatic-or-presymptomatic-spread/

University of Florida researchers find no asymptomatic or presymptomatic spread

Four researchers from the University of Florida Department of Biostatistics co-authored a study published online by the Journal of the American Medical Association. They performed a meta-analysis of 54 studies looking at the household secondary attack rate of SARS-CoV-2. According to the CDC, the secondary attack rate is the number of new cases among contacts divided by the total number of contacts.

…

The secondary attack rate for symptomatic index cases was 18.0% (95% CI 14.2%-22.1%), and the rate of asymptomatic and presymptomatic index cases was 0.7% (95% CI 0%-4.9%), "although there were few studies in the latter group."

The asymptomatic/presymptomatic secondary attack rate is not statistically different from zero, and the confidence interval is technically 0.7 ± 4.2, resulting in a range of -3.5%-4.9%, but attack rates cannot be negative, so it is truncated at 0

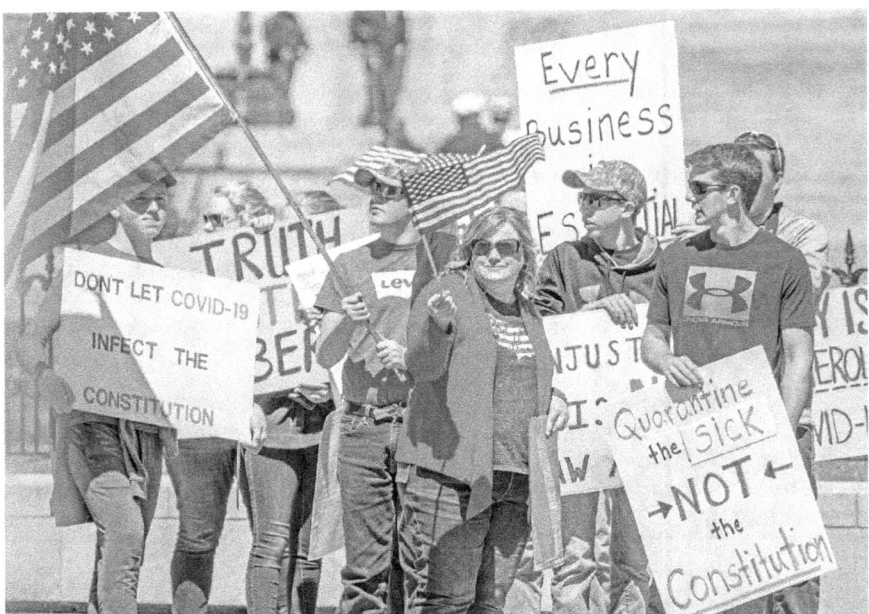
An anti-lockdown protest at the Ohio Statehouse in April 2020 amid the COVID-19 pandemic in the state.

'Irreparable damage': Over 6,000 scientists sign petition calling for end of coronavirus lockdowns[36]

| October 07, 2020 10:38 AM

==========

After supporting coronavirus lockdowns for months, the WHO just made the reversal of the year[37]

October 11th, 2020

---

[36] https://www.washingtonexaminer.com/news/irreparable-damage-over-6-000-scientists-sign-petition-calling-for-end-of-coronavirus-lockdowns
NOTE: the petition was ignored by politicians and health authorities
[37] https://bgr.com/2020/10/11/coronavirus-lockdown-world-health-organization-new-warning-covid-19/

> **Shutting Down Schools 'Makes Absolutely No Sense'**
> COVID-19 survival rates by age, posted by the CDC September 10, 2020:
>
> - Ages= birth to 19: 99.997%
> - Ages= 20 to 49: 99.98%
> - Ages= 50 to 69: 99.5%
> - Ages= 70 and up: 94.6%
>
> school-aged children from 5 to 17 years...there were 51 COVID-19 deaths reported in that age range from March 1 to September 10, 2020.
>
> "Now there are 56.4 million students in elementary, middle and high school in the United States so that means the chances by population, not by infection but by population, are less than 1 in a million per year for a student in school, and that's very important because we've shut down the schools in America, which causes a lot of problems," he said.
>
> every year more than 200 school-aged children, on average, die from the flu during a five-month flu season. "So, if you want to be consistent ... if you're going to close the schools for SARS-CoV-2 you must close them every year for the flu because it's actually much more severe in the school-age group."

As seen with the CDC admittance that the covid-19 death numbers they originally reported were wrong so too the continued use of the larger misleading number continues to be supported by the health officials, politicians and the media. Only 6% of the total number of deaths they initially reported as having supposedly died from "coronavirus" or "covid-19" disease was the truth, not 100%. So, 94% of people died, not from covid 19 disease alone but **WITH** co-morbid diseases, and only 4% without, Yet, the same high total numbers of supposed deaths from covid-19 disease continue to be used in the media, presumably to continue scaring the public. The fact that media messages are not being corrected by the CDC, FDA or government officials, points to, again, an ulterior motive, apparently to continue scaring people and prime them to obey officials and take **experimental gene and mind altering therapies** such as pseudo-vaccines and or implanted microchips as well as accept digital and chemical tagging, and tracking as well as financial control. So too here, with the reversed guidance of the WHO about lockdowns, the political authorities continued imposing them despite the change by the WHO, which they purport to be following. That continued use of a failed, if not more destructive policy, after being informed about it by the supposedly guiding institution points to an ulterior motive for its implementation other than science or good governance.

From Mind Control to Viruses: How the US Government Keeps Experimenting on Its Citizens[38]

By John W. Whitehead and Nisha Whitehead
Global Research, May 04, 2021

Many people are unaware or in denial of the sordid history of the US government experimentations on its own population. Consequently, they are also unable or unwilling to face the issue of their position as guinea pigs or cattle in the eyes of the power elites and their compromised and coerced technocratic servants (presidents, congress, corporate CEOs, and those manning the government agencies) that administer the experimentations on them. Thus, they are also unable to believe that the US Government and its agencies, meaning the people working in those agencies, would do such things as give them experimental substances while calling those experimental substances "approved and proven safe and effective", etc. Yet, the US Government and the people working in varied agencies have done just that and the indications are that the chemical gene therapies referred to as "vaccines" are also part of the deceptions that have been perpetrated throughout the history of the US government (especially in the 20th century and accelerating into the 21st century) and the fascistic relationship with businesses and corporations that is so ubiquitous as to be openly referred to as "private-public partnerships". "Private-public partnerships" are a euphemism for fascism. The definition of fascism is "collusion/cooperation/joining between corporations and government"; that union is invariably for the purpose of controlling and exploiting the population.

Dr. Pierre Kory MD.,[39] reviewed how the government agencies and the mainstream and social medias have sought to engage in specific tactics of deception to deceive the public into believing that there are no safe and effective drugs to prevent and or cure the disease referred to as "coronavirus" or "covid 19". He determined that a "DISINFORMATION PLAYBOOK" is in use involving the ignoring the positive proofs about the safety and effectiveness of the drug ivermectin for treating the disease

---

[38] https://www.globalresearch.ca/how-government-keeps-experimenting-citizens/5744256
Microchips In Our Brains - Big Tech's A.I. Agenda
https://www.youtube.com/watch?v=hpcam2IQ1h8
[39] https://www.youtube.com/watch?v=JzsRdcoW5kE

referred to as "coronavirus" or "covid 19". The disinformation playbook involves ignoring the trial results and confusing people, as the tobacco industry did, by ignoring positive trials and selecting trials that are designed to make the drug appear ineffective, at least to confuse people. These duplicitous techniques have and are being used in other industries as well, under the coordinated auspices of government agencies and corporations, in other words, fascism. A variety of tactics were used throughout the year 2020, that were perfected since the advent of the "public relations" (propaganda) industry and the deception techniques pioneered by the tobacco industry over the last century. The idea is to sow confusion through misunderstanding reinforced by misdirection and repeated propagandistic messages from politicians, celebrities and health officials. In this case, the idea is to dissuade people from knowing about or seeking out other alternatives to the experimental chemical gene therapies they want to foist on the population. By claiming that there are no other treatments the authorities can appear to be in compliance with the Nuremberg Treaty that says experimental treatments cannot be used when there are safe and effective treatments already available. The health authorities are also in violation of the Nuremberg Treaty because they are not giving full disclosure (informed consent) about the risks of the experimental vaccines. Another violation is saying that the experimental vaccines are safe and effective when the vaccine trial is only beginning so such a claim is baseless. These deception techniques work because the general public is ignorant and weak-willed as well as debilitated by unhealthy living, other drug use, and the psychological pressure from the fear-mongering and efforts to convince people that their "vaccine hesitancy" is based on unfounded concerns. On top of the aforesaid, there is also the issue of the built-in human predilection for following, obeying, and complying with authorities. So, debilitated people are being deceived and pressured by people who have in the past and are now perpetrating frauds on the population from positions of supposed authority. They use that authority now, through control of the media and having normalized the general cancel culture of all who espouse other points of view, to shut down any questioning of their positions and dictates, thereby preventing people from knowing about other opinions and answers to the problems of the society and the delusions that the leaders have perpetrated. The ignorance and weakness of the population allows the power elites to remain in power.

Dr. Wolfgang Wodarg on the 2009 Fake Pandemic and the Vaccination Scheme[40]

Dr. Wodarg: "I Think This Vaccination is Really the Pinnacle of the Crime"

Dr. Wolfgang Wodarg: One of the Most Important Experts the World Should Hear About[41]

---

[40] https://www.weblyf.com/2021/01/dr-wolfgang-wodarg-on-the-2009-fake-pandemic-and-the-vaccination-scheme/
https://gatesofvienna.net/2020/11/dr-wodarg-i-think-this-vaccination-is-really-the-pinnacle-of-the-crime/
[41] https://www.weblyf.com/2020/12/dr-wolfgang-wodarg-one-of-the-most-important-experts-the-world-should-hear-about/

Safe and Effective Drug and Supplement Alternatives to Vaccines Ignored and Denied by Health Officials with Support from Mainstream Media-Despite the Proofs of Their Efficacy

A few countries have started to accept, or we may say started to suppress information less and refuse the truth of science less, that there are effective supplements and medicines to prevent or heal from coronavirus disease (covid 19), like Vitamin D3 and C, Astralagus, Melatonin, Zinc and drugs like Hydroxychloroquine[42] and Ivermectin. These supplements and medicines have been proven to be effective in prevention and cure of the disease Covid-19 from the supposed coronavirus; still, most medical agencies of most countries actively neglect advocating these supplements and drugs and or discourage, prohibit and or refuse to accept them (suppress or deny, in the face of evidence) and rather continue searching and advocating for expensive drugs or more "experimental chemical therapies" or "gene therapies" or "genetic engineering" that cannot be considered as "vaccines", but yet are promoted as such. It turns out that a strong motive to suppress and ignore the known, safe and effective drugs is because according to regulations, if there are safe and effective treatments for a disease, it is not allowed to implement experimental unproven therapies like the experimental chemical gene therapies that are being referred to as "vaccines".

---

[42] https://aapsonline.org/hcq-90-percent-chance/

COVID-19 mRNA Shots Are Legally Not Vaccines
Analysis by Dr. Joseph Mercola[43]

So, with the evidence growing about the nature of the lower lethality of the virus and the safe and effective supplements and drug therapies available to handle it, why do governments and certain non-governmental institutions around the world continue to advocate the use of therapies, protocols, and mandates that do not have scientific evidence to support them and have the opposite effect of the goals stated by those same institutions and authorities? Why are persons in positions of power, such as Anthony Fauci[44] and Dr. Tedros Adhanom Ghebreyesus[45] at the World Health Organization, who apparently have serious conflicts of interest and serious allegations of corruption, allowed to head the most powerful policy directing positions in global health? Why are presidents and prime ministers, the world over, and in concert, so willing to impose unscientific, unproven, and demonstrably injurious mandates on their populations, destroying their own country's economies? The implications to the answers of the seemingly rhetorical questions above are the key areas for reflection that are enjoined in this book.

TOOLS FOR COERCIVE PSYCHOLOGICAL CONDITIONING AND THE WILLINGNESS TO USE THEM

Facemasks, lockdowns, school closures, and business closures, all supposedly for "public safety", have the effect of not reducing infections but instead promote increasing poverty and suffering while also training the population to obey authority while quelling protests under the guise of protecting people by preventing gatherings. By accusing those who question their actions as spreading "fake news", the authorities and the

---

[43] https://articles.mercola.com/sites/articles/archive/2021/02/09/coronavirus-mrna-vaccine.aspx?ui=152220df1deda081f73727bc10a8407027b248ba493a7ce71f4a1e73a6c1d882&sd=20200829&cid_source=dnl&cid_medium=email&cid_content=art1HL&cid=20210209_HL2&mid=DM799847&rid=1080024489

[44] National Institute of Allergy and Infectious Diseases
The Covid-19 Pandemic as a Psychological Coup d'Etat
https://thegarynullshow.podbean.com/e/the-gary-null-show-012521/

[45] WHO Director-General
https://ecadforum.com/2017/04/23/dr-tedros-adhanom-is-an-individual-suspected-of-a-crime-against-humanity/

media promote fear with "Orwellian"[46] psychological conditioning carefully crafted phrases and slogans, like "stay home, stay safe," "if you love your parents lock them up," "to visit each other is to kill each other," "keep your distance, wash your hands, think of others," "build back better," "the new normal." <u>The patterns of the phrases usually have three and are repeated in groups of threes:</u> this is by design, as a proven technique of the "rule of three" in psychological conditioning. These are specially chosen phrases that turn into memes and buzzwords that convey feelings and concepts that come into vogue and can consciously and subliminally support social trends. When repeatedly stated, as is done by politicians and the mass media, the slogans and coercive statements become implanted as thoughts influencing behavior in the population. They build in the mind and take on the quality of "truths" that are <u>not</u> true but that people come to believe as truths that are proven or accepted realities but which are, in actuality, only supported by the emotion of fear backed up by ignorance if not outright delusions that people will defend even to the extent of a physical altercation against those who may hold a difference of opinion or even present contrary evidences.

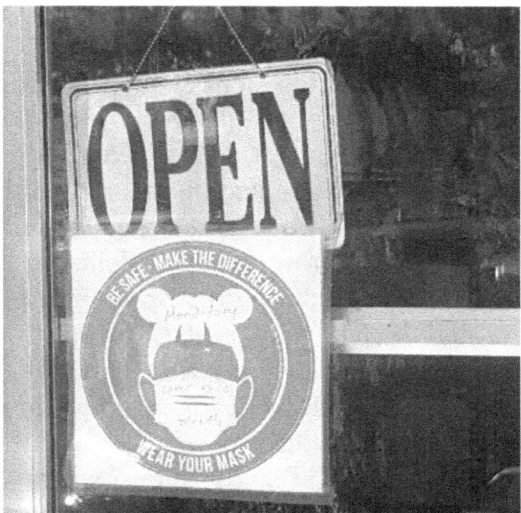

Example of a store door entrance showing the blind belief in the statements by authorities forcing the wearing of masks that have been scientifically found to make no statistical difference in infection rates. It is a useless gesture as far as promoting health but useful in promoting and maintaining fear and disease.

---

[46] https://youtu.be/pa6LszZa7pg International best-selling author, Dr Vernon Coleman MB ChB DSc FRSA, explains how governments have used mind control techniques to manipulate us during this alleged crisis.

The audio-visual media such as supposed television newscasters and reporters reinforce the propaganda lies by wearing face masks even when they are in the middle of a street with nobody around, to "set an example"[47], even though the arbitrary social distancing regulation is to wear a mask when it is not possible to be 6 feet or more between oneself and others. The mask-wearing regulation was made up from the start, with no scientific evidence. This factor has been known since before the year 2020 and subsequent studies in 2020 and now in 2021 have confirmed the uselessness of mask-wearing for the general asymptomatic public. Yet, facemasks are still being pushed even for people who have received the experimental gene therapy drugs referred to as "vaccines".

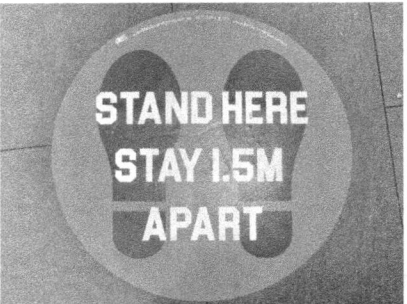

Above: Social distancing signs at shops in Brisbane.

The image above is an example of a useless floor sign, similar to many around the world, immediately adopted by businesses that are advancing the false idea of keeping the arbitrary (no science behind it) distance from everyone else and thereby fostering fear and delusion. Social distancing never worked when it was tried during the Spanish FLU pandemic of the early 20th century, and is just another task people are told to do to supposedly help themselves but which in reality debilitate and cause disease and supports the **FEAR APPEAL** tactic, imposed by the authorities, along with submission to the "authorities" that are issuing the arbitrary rules. People must realize that, as the MIT study below confirms, the science does not support masks, social distancing, or lockdowns and there is no safe distance while living in a society of human animals except good nutrition, exercise, sunshine along with the safe and effective supplements and drugs proven to either promote a healthy immune system and or cure the disease referred to as covid 19.

---

[47] https://articles.mercola.com/sites/articles/archive/2021/05/22/covid-mask-theater-caught-on-camera.aspx?ui=152220df1deda081f73727bc10a8407027b248ba493a7ce71f4a1e73a6c1d882&sd=20200829&cid_source=dnl&cid_medium=email&cid_content=art2HL&cid=20210522&mid=DM891109&rid=1164262547

MIT researchers say you're no safer from Covid indoors at 6 feet or 60 feet in new study challenging social distancing policies[48]

As introduced earlier, the fraudulent supposed newscasters and reporters are being paraded by the mainstream media to "model" "good behavior" and encouraging "compliance" with "authorities" but in reality, they are reinforcing the fear and delusion set up by those "authorities" along with misunderstanding the mask-wearing policy as they shirk their responsibility to investigate the truth about the false security of mask-wearing, social-distancing or lockdowns and pass on the ideal of blind obedience by their words and actions. Thereby they are misleading the public and fomenting more fear and hysteria about a falsified pandemic and the true means to promote health and wellbeing. There is neither necessity nor any scientific justification for wearing masks alone in the middle of the street supposedly to protect oneself from a virus. In fact, there is no evidence that wearing any mask helps prevent getting infected by any given virus. Instead, they model obedience, compliance, and uncritical thinking for the population; so, instead of being investigative journalists, the media has become, instead, stenographers and repeaters of what they are told to say through the corporate policies sent to them by the power elite owners of the media companies. In this context, the term "presstitutes" which has been used to describe the mainstream media, would seem to be very apt indeed. In that context, the mainstream media supposed news reporters have become sycophants of and stenographers for the power elites and their technocratic bought-off politicians. Some may claim, however, that the modeling being done by politicians and media personalities is for encouraging compliance for the public good. Others point out that mainstream media admits to pushing the covid story and modeling behaviors to raise ratings and make more money.

---

[48] https://www.cnbc.com/2021/04/23/mit-researchers-say-youre-no-safer-from-covid-indoors-at-6-feet-or-60-feet-in-new-study.html

CNN staffer tells Project Veritas network played up COVID-19 death toll for ratings[49]

By Emily Jacobs April 14, 2021

==========

CNN technical director admits to pushing COVID panic and using death tracker to do it by Andrew Mark Miller | April 14, 2021

When does the "innocent" desire to encourage good actions, in others, turn into an act that is used for coercion and intimidation to promote conformity with a social policy that is fraudulent? Answer: when the reason for doing it has been divorced from reason, rationality, goodwill, and truth; when it is an encouragement being done by someone who wants to do it not because they believe in it but because they want to keep their job; when it is being pushed not based on science or evidence but someone's profit, or conjecture or whim or delusion or "power trip".

When does a political act take on the format of conspiracy? When almost all of the politicians and the media personalities start saying the same slogans and phrases, they model the same behaviors when they are in public but not necessarily in private, and start enacting the same or similar policies or supporting such policies in concert. It is not necessary to have a classical conspiracy where all the conspirators sit around a table and all agree to take the same actions at the same time. People or organizations can act in lockstep without being in contact with each other because they have the same values or are equally corrupt and equally interested in the same corrupt goals that they have been allowed to practice, as an industry. An example of the latter case is the mainstream media companies that pushed lies to get higher ratings and in so doing are also serving the ulterior motives of their power elite owners. In a hierarchical society, such as is found in most of the world corporations and governments, and especially in oligarchic plutocracy systems like the USA and other countries, the dictates coming from the top to bottom in a series of successively powerless (cannot

---

[49] https://nypost.com/2021/04/14/cnn-staffer-tells-project-veritas-network-played-up-covid-19-death-toll-for-ratings/

refuse orders from their superiors under penalty of loss of employment) successions of management levels.

Accordingly, the real owners and directors issue orders to underlying managers who control the workforce of the government agency or corporation. Then those managers and sub-managers carry out the orders even if they are unfair or seem irrational to the goal of good governance, good business practices, and or ethical conscience. They follow orders under penalty of firing. So the orders are distributed to the technocrats and agency and corporate managers, to be carried out under penalty of firing and loss of income, with the true desired outcome of the policies being unknown to them but only to the real owners and directors at the top, who collude and support policies that are meant to achieve goals other than good governance and the welfare of the population as a whole.[50] Therefore, the force in an inverted totalitarian fascist police state is not primarily or at least initially with violence but under threat of loss of income. So currency and livelihood are the main items threatened through the coercion and intimidation tool (fiat currency) of the power elite. This coercion operates on political leaders and managers of government agencies and corporate managers as well as the general population. Thus, keeping the middle managers and general population under constant stress and fear over loss of livelihood and at the same time maintaining general employment income with only subsistence-level wages, relative to the cost of living, is an important component for having and maintaining coercive leverage over the middle managers and general population of the society.

It is well known that humans are susceptible to the feelings, opinions, actions, and reactions of others as a basis for developing their feelings, opinions, behaviors, and actions. Dishonest leaders seek to control the feelings and behaviors of the population in order to promote opinions, thoughts, and actions they want in the population; they do this not out of altruism or goodwill but out of a sociopathic and egoistic need for control of others for their own (the power elite and the appointed leaders and their employed managers) benefit. The dishonest leaders use misdirections such as distractions with identity politics, race conflict, social issues, etc. to redirect mistrust and anger away from the true source behind the apparently irrational, destructive, divisive, and warmongering policies, towards segments or groups within the population. The misdirection operates through the speeches of politicians and it is echoed in the media. Another

---

[50] https://www.corbettreport.com/how-can-a-global-conspiracy-work-questions-for-corbett-074/

primary method of misdirection is by confusion, that is, issuing contradictory policies or calling allegations of misconduct, malfeasance, or incompetence as "conspiracy theories" or labeling criticisms of the power elite establishment policies as "fake news" or "unpatriotic" or putting out completely fabricated counter-narratives to foment confusion in the minds of listeners. An example of this was the introduction of actual false research, in supposedly prestigious journals, about the drug hydroxychloroquine with false evidence about its safety so as to discourage its use and force people to wait for the expensive drugs and vaccines. Yet, after it was discovered that this was indeed fake news with an ulterior motive, the media continued fomenting the false narrative about its deadly effects instead of the correct information about its benefit for healing from covid-19 disease.

Covid-19: Lancet retracts paper that halted hydroxychloroquine trials[51]

Lancet Formally Retracts Fake Hydroxychloroquine Study Used By Media To Attack Trump[52]

June 4, 2020

The decades-long corruption of politics that foments division and intolerance, that accelerated with the republican revolution of the 1990s is the kneejerk reaction to repudiate anything said or proposed by the opposing political party, regardless of if it is true, right, or useful. The idea is to ideologically oppose the other because they are not one of you. This irrational and psychologically deficient way of relating fostered a toxic social-cultural environment that came to a fever pitch during the 2016 presidential election that was won by Donald Trump. A serial liar, sexist, racist, and crass personality, Trump began to realize that Hydroxychloroquine was useful against the coronavirus disease and that Anthony Fauci was doing gain of function research to produce more pathogenic viruses. Trump sought to speak out about hydroxychloroquine and distance himself from and reduce the prominence of Fauci. Yet, the

---

[51] https://www.theguardian.com/world/2020/jun/04/covid-19-lancet-retracts-paper-that-halted-hydroxychloroquine-trials
[52] https://thefederalist.com/2020/06/04/lancet-formally-retracts-fake-hydroxychloroquine-study-used-by-media-to-attack-trump-inbox/

bought and paid for news media and democrat politicians opposed anything he said, no matter who got hurt by not getting the life-saving drug. So, the degraded political climate fostered by the population and their politicians and the acceptance by the population of a vulgar pathological liar suffering from narcissistic psychological disorder led to a scenario where power elite personalities in banks and drug corporations saw the opportunity to discredit Trump and his idea of hydroxychloroquine and in so doing delay people's use of the drug until lucrative tools of control, the experimental chemical gene therapies referred to as "vaccines," could be brought to market. This is how the corruption of the culture itself leads to its political self-delusion and scientific blindness that causes its own suffering; this is largely due to the allowance of degraded cultural ideals and ideologies, such as racism, sexism, identity politics, and capitalism to corrupt the politics of the society. The term "allowance" is used here because the society itself, the people, and the leaders they allow to be in positions of leadership, are the ones accepting and allowing the acceptable social interactions, ideals, and ideologies that define the society. Such is the fate of a society that becomes degraded due to failing to live by truth in its culture, politics and economics.

The above mentioned issues are compounded by the innate human psychological weaknesses that can be exploited by sociopathic personalities. An example of the digital age enhancements to the program of mass population control have been advanced through the Facebook, university researchers and Department of Defense partnership for mind-control. Such partnerships, coupled with the fear appeal techniques and Milgram Experiment[53] evidence of human compliance to authority, and the propaganda machine of mainstream and social media form a powerful and unprecedented society-wide inescapable digital bubble of control that permeates the entire society.

Facebook mind control experiments linked to DoD research on civil unrest[54]
2 Jul, 2014

---

[53] https://nature.berkeley.edu/ucce50/ag-labor/7article/article35.htm
[54] https://www.rt.com/usa/169848-pentagon-facebook-study-minerva/

Facebook reveals news feed experiment to control emotions
Sun 29 Jun 2014

PRESIDENTS, PRIME MINISTERS AS LIGHTNING RODS TO DISTRACT POPULATIONS.

The president, prime minister, etc. positions in politics serve as a focus for hope as well as the anger of the population, that looks to such persons as responsible for the way things are instead of looking at the persons who are really pulling the strings behind the government and private institutional policies of society and the divisiveness, the support of demagogues, media propaganda and censorship, the promotion of disease, wars, fossil fuels based economy, etc. Varied problems of humanity have simple solutions *if* there were a capacity and willingness to live by the truth. However, a society guided by truth would not allow the power elites to remain in power. It is noteworthy that humanity can fly to the moon but cannot improve the medical system or organize a simple and efficient method to get a driver's license renewed. It is also noteworthy that throughout history there have been apparent good policies and laws that over time are changed by other laws or withdrawn, by incoming political rulers in favor of other policies that were touted as better but in reality have the mission of demolishing the previously existing better policy or law. This is a well-known tactic that produces a situation wherein people think there has been progress, but on balance, the progress is minimal or relatively nil. This means that while progress appears to have occurred: there are more people with healthcare now than before, there are more people that have modern conveniences than before, etc. In reality, those modern conveniences that have been allowed to reach the general public, have not improved life substantially above the quality of life of the past generations especially in comparison to the quality of life of the power elites but do serve as distractors away from true progress and real quality of life that should not be defined in terms of the number of conveniences and or material goods that one can acquire. Some example is the more stressed, more complexed, more polluted, more vaccinated, drug and social media addicted nature of modern society. Can these issues be said to contribute to a greater quality of life now than what a person experienced a generation or two ago, even if we consider that their life expectancy, in the previous generation, was lower?[55] Another example of the contradiction of the appearance of health is the recent finding of the reversal of the life expectancy index.

So, what appeared to be progress and improvement in life expectancy led to a reversal; on balance it is neutral or lower but yet serves as an illusion of doing better. Actually, even as the life expectancy grew longer, in nominal terms, it was fraught with greater stress, more disease, and in reality diminishing wealth and quality of life all along. Also, all along, that situation wherein the population is managed into endless hamster wheel living, serfdom, and cannon fodder value, served the purpose of the enrichment of the power elite as their policies helped to dupe people into believing they were progressing even as they supported the loss of wealth, the propaganda, the warmongering and toxic lifestyle choices they were allowed to choose from. Meaning: If people only have choices allowed by the power elites then their idea that they have choices is an illusion that serves the personalities that allowed them to choose between those choices. EXAMPLE: The delusion of choice works in terms of political choices between two sets of politicians that speak seemingly different rhetoric but who will both follow the dictates of the power elites that paid for their campaigns and will pay for their execution if they deviate from the power elite plans; EXAMPLE: this works in terms of being given the choice between using fossil fuels or renewables that will not be allowed to compete with fossil fuels. These are illusory choices that cannot be considered as choices at all. Therefore, the program of implementing seemingly irrational policies that appear to be "wrong" to a rational or ethical person and yet are implemented anyway, necessarily fomenting decades of disease, social strife and struggle in the purposely corrupt political morass to get changed, and never-improving social institutions and bloating inefficient bureaucracies will remain in force. Another example of the relative context of capitalist fascism leading to impending neo-feudalism is that while the horrors of chattel slavery and indentured servitude, of some societies in previous generations was barbarous and abhorrent, the new power elite plan of digital currencies will digitally enslave ALL people, worldwide, who belong to the non-power elite class (power elite absolute control of money, media, livelihood, personal freedom, etc.).

The dishonest leaders put up their technocratic representatives (political leaders and managers of government agencies and corporate managers) to

---

[55] Note: in recent years the trend of increasing life expectancy has revered and the present generation has a lower life expectancy that the previous.

implement the policies, which includes using the media for propaganda, censorship and playing audiovisual subtle and some not so subtle cues that "encourage" people to develop certain opinions and desires that will lead to certain desired feelings and actions that are in accord with the designs of the power elite's plan for them. The psychological conditioning theme has been researched and additional scientifically outlined methods of coercion and intimidation have been delineated, including giving controlled, subjugated people supposed actions to do to mitigate that fear such as mask-wearing, social distancing, etc. This is done so they may think they are doing something to help themselves and at the same time show compliance with the supposed goal of collective wellbeing. In actuality, they are not promoting wellbeing but rather disease and stress which debilitates them and solidifies their subservience to the supposed authorities. That subservience to the authorities trains the population to behave in ways that are approved by the supposed authorities, thereby ceding autonomy and sovereignty to the power elites and their minions.

MEDICAL TYRANNY AS A TOOL OF THE POWER ELITES

The usurpation of power and the application of that power based on supposed medical expertise and or a supposed emergency supposedly due to a disease or pandemic may be referred to as **"medical tyranny"** or **"medical mafia"** or **"medical fascism."** When coupled with cooperation by government officials and the mainstream media this "medical tyranny" or "medical mafia" may be referred to as "medical fascism". Examples of medical tyranny can range from a nurse telling a parent they will call the police, have them arrested and have the child taken away due to child abuse for not getting them vaccinated, to coercing a nurse to take vaccines or otherwise barring them from working at a hospital, or barring children from school, that are not vaccinated, to forcing people to accept vaccinations or otherwise not being able to travel, keep a job or use public facilities, etc.

This medical tyranny presupposes that there is an absolute right that officials can confer upon themselves if there is a "public medical emergency". Before ceding their sovereign right to their own bodily integrity to anyone else, conscientious persons need to consider the following issues for themselves as individuals and the risks to themselves and to society if their rights are handed to unethical sociopathic personalities.

- ✓ Who determines what is a "public medical emergency"?
- ✓ Who determines what and when a "public medical emergency" is in effect?
- ✓ Who should be the ones determining what to do about a "public medical emergency"?
- ✓ <u>Even if there was an actual (true) "public medical emergency"</u> is it right for only supposed medical personnel, many of whom have been demonstrated to have presently and in the past, conflicts of interest, errors or criminality to be the arbiters of what actions should be taken?
- ✓ <u>Even if there was a real (true) "public medical emergency"</u> is it right for only the supposed medical personnel, who clearly have conflicts of interest, biases, and have been misleading people about the dangers of "vaccines" in general and never talk about vitamins and nutrition to bolster the immune system?
- ✓ <u>Even if there was a real (true) "public medical emergency"</u> is it right to have non-medical persons such as Bill Gates,[56] who have been demonstrated to have rapacious interests in vaccines and desires for secret depopulation, eugenics, genocide or have distributed on unapproved vaccines that killed or damaged thousands of people around the world or have stated they want to use vaccines to reduce the world populations, especially, though not limited to concentrating on non-white populations and or have criminal backgrounds, to be the arbiters of what actions should be taken?

In reality, the right was self-given, by the so-called officials, to themselves and was not granted by law or certified by public choice through elections. Therefore, their self-granted authority is an authoritarian/totalitarian act that purposefully circumvents the sovereignty and human rights of people. Thus, the medical establishment can neither be trusted nor relied upon to, on their own, righteously use an absolute medical power since they themselves are caught up in the delusion of their absolute correctness and are compromised

---

[56] BILL GATES AMERICAS SELF-APPOINTED VACCINE CZAR
https://garynull.com/bill-gates-america_s-self-appointed-vaccine-czar-prn/
BILL GATES BLASTED AS "VACCINE CRIMINAL" IN ITALIAN PARLIAMENT
https://thenewamerican.com/bill-gates-blasted-as-vaccine-criminal-in-italian-parliament/
BILL GATES FUNDS COVERT VACCINE NANOTECHNOLOGY
http://gna.squarespace.com/home/bill-gates-funds-covert-vaccine-nanotechnology.html
WHO IS BILL GATES? (FULL DOCUMENTARY, 2020)
https://www.corbettreport.com/who-is-bill-gates-full-documentary-2020/
BILL GATES AND THE POPULATION CONTROL GRID
https://www.corbettreport.com/?s=bill+gates

by the same human failings as anyone else, self-righteousness, desire for wealth, power, prestige, etc. that blinds them from seeing their own shortcomings, corruption or errors.

FEAR APPEAL AS A TOOL OF SOCIOPATHIC POWER ELITE TYRANTS

Fauci Wants You Scared, Anxious, and Compliant– It's Scientific!
By Ginger Ross Breggin and Peter R. Breggin M.D.[57]
November 06, 2020

Tyrannical psychological conditioning techniques have been well defined under a public health concept called "Fear Appeal" (i.e. how to scare people for the purpose of controlling them) is a specific psychological motivation technique used to affect populations through fear.[58] "Fear Appeal" requires making the source of fear personal and then giving people something to do about it like wearing masks. "Fear Appeal" is not concerned with civil rights or personal human rights; it is authoritarian, based on the idea that the public health officials know what is right so they supposedly have the right to impose their policies in a totalitarian manner.

The Fear Appeal leads to confusion, rises to anxiety, and culminates in a state of helplessness. In this way the psychological state of the populace can be conditioned into helplessness wherein people live fearfully and sufficiently psychologically and physically weakened so much to accept suffering and stress that can be relieved through a "new normal" that is less hopeful, less free and less abundant than the previous state; i.e. destroy the economy and foment mass impoverishment and suffering followed by people accepting a standard of living that is below the previous one. Stressed, fearful, and anxious people will do what they are told to do regardless of if it makes sense or not and they will gladly accept what they are given just for the opportunity to relieve the anxiety, even if it means accepting a lower standard of living, a "new normal". So, "Fear Appeal" is an important contrivance used to produce the desired compromised psychological state is that is ideal for social manipulation.

---

[57] https://breggin.com/fauci-wants-you-scared-anxious-and-compliant-its-scientific/
[58] The Link Between Fear Appeal and COVID-19 Perception- Interview With Dr. Peter Breggin https://youtu.be/iTr1BOdaDxU

FEAR APPEAL AS A TOOL FOR MANIPULATION OF THE PUBLIC INTO CULT BEHAVIORS[59]

Thus, the immoral and unethical technique of "Fear Appeal" may be thought of as a formalized, well researched, and scientifically honed "Orwellian"/"Brave New World" sociopathic psychological extension of a totalitarian control method for social conditioning. The fear appeal may also be thought of as a guiding manipulative tactic in support of the philosophy (control) behind the purpose for the use of propaganda, censorship, and misdirection of the public away from the human power elite source of strife in society and towards focusing on presidents, prime ministers, and governors or the neighbor next door who refuses to wear a mask as "the problem" causing unrest and disease in the society. As a tool it is another specialized method of coercion and intimidation, to be added to the other established ones that may be more forceful and directly confrontational, such as the use of the police and or army. The Fear Appeal has been a contributing factor in the development of a society-wide "covidmania" or "covidmania cult" that irrationally and unquestioningly follows the cult leaders (health authorities, political authorities, media authorities) of the covid pandemic fraud.[60] In this context, the covidmania cult members are those who believe, unquestioningly, the dictates of politicians, heads of the health agencies, and the media while disbelieving anyone who says anything that contradicts them even when showing evidence that those supposed "authorities" are either ignorant, wrong, contradicting themselves, lying or are demonstrably otherwise sociopathic, psychotic, corrupt, criminal and or unethical, immoral or untrustworthy. The people, who are the followers of the cult leaders, still believe despite evidence and continue acting in a delusional and even psychotic manner to their own detriment. They may also readily attack anyone who contradicts their beliefs or the dictates of the cult leaders. The cult followers also refuse to recognize that supposed cult leaders are being controlled by tacit manipulators, the power elites such as the Bill Gateses and Klaus Schwabses of the world. Another component of "covidmania" or the "covidmania cult" are the cult following health workers, the nurses, and the doctors who are indiscriminately administering the untested, unproven and

---

[59] https://articles.mercola.com/sites/articles/archive/2020/11/15/how-is-fear-appeal-used-in-public-health-messaging.aspx?cid_source=youtube&cid_medium=video&cid=articles_the-link-between-fear-appeal-and-covid-19-perception-interview-with-dr-peter-breggin
[60] https://www.bitchute.com/video/cWCE1h0ZMk4g/
https://www.bitchute.com/video/rTPzMkTAxQOH/

evidently poisonous, and dangerous experimental chemical gene therapies referred to as "vaccines." They too are not questioning the dictates of their superiors as they also chant the mantra of "vaccines are safe and effective" that they were told to believe and repeat, even as the new, untested, unproven, experimental covid chemical gene therapies referred to as "vaccines" have, so far, killed and maimed more people than all the other vaccines in the prior 10 or more years.[61] Additionally, the same cult following health workers, the nurses and the doctors who are part of the cult of believing in vaccines unquestioningly, are not doing their due diligence fulfilling their responsibility to inform the people they are injecting that the chemical gene therapies referred to as "vaccines" are an experiment and that they will be guinea pigs in the experiment that lasts for at least 2 years. Instead they and the media and the politicians lie by saying the chemical injections are safe and effective even though the experimental period of the vaccine trial, does not end for 2 more years. Instead they to quash any information about that issue or questioning the theories behind the vaccines; instead they all try to censor information in their institutions (hospitals, health agencies) and in the media, about the vaccine experiment, the true absolute efficacy (1%, not 90% as was promoted) and its dangers.

FEAR APPEAL AND THE "NEW NORMAL" MEME

The "new normal" meme is in reality a tightened totalitarian police and surveillance state, but now in a context of a changed, impoverished economic reality. Hence, the idea of a "Great Currency Reset", is also, in the midst of the supposed pandemic crisis, now being promoted at large. The supposed monetary great reset is an economic condition whereby the currency that has been so debased by the power elite malfeasance[62] is in need of "resetting," to be discontinued, terminated, and deprecated. It is to have its value reset along with a move from paper to digital currency, that will supposedly solve the problem of the collapsing currency (US dollar) and the US economy that was already on track to leave people in a lesser (impoverished due to inflation) economically viable state anyway. The continuing devaluation and inevitable demise of the US dollar, due to regular inflation and added currency creation (bailouts and quantitative easing) by the central banks, in its current form, has worldwide implications that will leave its users worldwide more impoverished, if not

---

[61] Dr. Vernon Coleman   https://brandnewtube.com/v/fRdX4T
Dr. John Bergman   www.drbvip.com/
[62] See the books: *Malfeasance and Immorality* and *Collapse of Civilization* by Dr. Muata Ashby

destitute. In turn, the holders of valuable assets such as real estate or gold or those who would be the first users of whatever the new currency would be would become more enriched. Such a worldwide upheaval would be more acceptable if it is explained as a result of the supposed virus caused economic collapse instead of it is recognized that the collapse was already underway and caused by the same power elite that enacted the malfeasance and directed the unnecessary lockdowns and is proposing solutions to "solve" the problem that the banks and politicians created in the first place. So, the banks and politicians created the problems with the currency by engaging in malfeasance and the recent economic crash and impending world economic collapse were accelerated <u>not by the virus but by the purposeful action of imposing unnecessary lockdowns on the population and providing "free currency" bailouts to banks and wall street companies</u>. The concern, by those who are not operating under fear or reactionary emotions, is that the solutions proffered by the power elite will be more of the same kinds of economic policies that enrich the power elite and impoverish everyone else. Many have sought refuge from this impending reset of the currency, in hard assets like real estate, precious metals and crypto currencies, both of which are expected to at least hold their value through the upcoming reset and social/political crisis that will likely ensue.

Meanwhile, as the government has imposed the fraud of corona virus scaring and false policies to supposedly help the situation, the government and financial sectors have colluded (fascism) to have more financial malfeasance in the economy (giving free money to pharmaceutical companies for chemical chemo therapies called "vaccines" and more bailouts to companies and banks) that result in economic bubbles such as the increasing unsustainable housing costs and the inflated stock and bond markets that will lead to collapse as previous bubbles have. When the bubbles burst, that will lead to greater impoverishment of the population but those who received the currency first[63] (a phenomenon called "cantillon effect) and purchased hard assets of real value will retain that wealth as others still in the markets, will suffer devastating losses. Now that malfeasance has accelerated, with the Federal Reserve central bank printing more money for bailouts to give banks and corporations more currency to acquire more real assets, those assets and wealth will continue to be further out of reach for the general population. Dr. Peter Breggin, Psychiatrist, made an assessment of the power elite imposing the coronavirus lockdowns,

---

[63] Those who get to use the money first are the banks and the corporations associated with them – all of which are owned by the power elites.

mask wearing and social distancing as a concerted plan against the population.

Fauci-Funded Chinese/US Research Led to COVID-19
All Suspicions Confirmed
The Chinese government now has the unlimited ability to keep manufacturing pandemic viruses
By Peter R. Breggin MD and Ginger Breggin[64]
September, 18, 2020

Dr. Fauci's COVID-19 Treachery with Chilling Ties to the Chinese Military
by Peter R. Breggin MD & Ginger R. Breggin[65]
October 19, 2020

What can be done to counteract the fear-mongering politicians, corrupt public health officials and corrupt mainstream media?

- ✓ Seek the truth in alternative information sources.
- ✓ Participate with others who are seeking truth.
- ✓ Apply the true information and reject the lies.
- ✓ Affirm truth in the silence of internal reflection and also when asked by those who are experiencing fear and anxiety.
- ✓ Participate and cooperate with others who are making efforts to live by truth.
- ✓ Seek out and practice sound money economics such saving, investing in real assets such as land and precious metals.
- ✓ Prepare for the impending collapse of society by becoming more self-sufficient.

---

[64] https://myaccount.ingramspark.com/?stp=%2fTitles%2fTitleSearch
[65] https://breggin.com/dr-faucis-covid-19-treachery/

THE FRAUD OF VACCINES AND VACCINES AS TOOLS OF THE POWER ELITES, MEDICAL TYRANNY AND PROFITS

Vaccines are touted as being the cause of the reduction in human diseases. Also, they are touted as safe and effective therapies. Firstly, there is evidence that many drugs and vaccines were failures and withdrawn/recalled after being approved and then killing and maiming many people.[66] If vaccines are safe and effective what is the need of recalling them? Were they not touted as safe and effective when they were first introduced? The last major vaccine debacle was the Swine Flu vaccine of 1976.[67]

Those vaccines that are touted as successful were introduced at a time when general society-wide hygiene was improved and the diseases that the vaccines were created for were already in decline due to the better hygiene of the society; then the credit for the reduction was given to the vaccines and not to the better hygiene.

The placebo controlled randomized study is seen as the "gold standard" proof of safety and efficacy. So, the *inert placebo*-controlled double-blind randomized study is regarded as the highest scientific testing protocol to determine if any treatment safe and is truly useful in achieving the desired or expected goal of helping and or curing a disease. There is no vaccine that has been proven to be safe and effective, for any given person, using a gold standard placebo controlled randomized study.[68] Why have there been no placebo controlled randomized studies done on vaccines? If vaccines are safe and effective why did the US congress need to pass a law, in 1986, saying that no one can sue the vaccine drug companies for any death or injury that the vaccines may cause? Answer: because the results show that vaccines are not safe and effective for any given person, nor are they effective for increasing health or preventing disease. Also, it would be discovered that vaccines do more damage than the diseases and that healthy living and natural supplements and real safe drugs are more effective; thus drug companies would lose income by the exposure of the obvious failure and dangers of vaccines and drug therapies.

---

[66] www.cdc.gov/vaccines/pubs/pinkbook/downloads/appendices/B/discontinued_vaccines.pdf
https://en.wikipedia.org/wiki/List_of_withdrawn_drugs
[67] https://www.latimes.com/archives/la-xpm-2009-apr-27-sci-swine-history27-story.html
[68] https://www.bitchute.com/video/y9UnRNlLwznP/

The desired next phase of politics and economics, by the power elite, is one that will force more people into poverty willingly while transferring more wealth to and leaving fewer (reduced population) people wealthy and with power to control their lives. The fear about the supposed virus pandemic has been used as an excuse to impose business closings that are leading to impoverishment. Along the way, the imposed "new fear normal" way of life facilitates willing acceptance of things people would not otherwise accept such as "experimental chemical gene therapies" surreptitiously referred to as "vaccines" which do not meet the definition of a vaccine. Again, vaccines, in general, have never been proven to be safe and effective for any given individual and have not been proven to be safe or effective via a gold standard using an inert placebo-controlled double-blind trial method. The new current "experimental chemical gene therapies", for covid 19, passed off as vaccines, such as those that use experimental mRNA technology, which also have never been proven to work even in animals, is being accepted widely by many people even as, as of the date of this writing (May. 2021) tens of thousands of people have died and been injured after taking those "experimental chemical therapies", while the drug companies that produce them reap great financial rewards, with no legal liability for any injuries they may cause.

> https://www.cdc.gov/vaccines/covid-19/info-by-product/clinical-considerations.html#Appendix-B
>
> **Interim Clinical Considerations for Use of mRNA COVID-19 Vaccines Currently Authorized in the United States**
>
> *Contraindications*
>
> CDC considers a history of the following to be a contraindication to vaccination with both the Pfizer-BioNTech and Moderna COVID-19 vaccines:
>
> - Severe allergic reaction (e.g., anaphylaxis) after a previous dose of an mRNA COVID-19 vaccine or any of its components
> - Immediate allergic reaction of any severity to a previous dose of an mRNA COVID-19 vaccine or any of its components (including polyethylene glycol [PEG])*
> - Immediate allergic reaction of any severity to polysorbate (due to potential cross-reactive hypersensitivity with the vaccine ingredient PEG)*
>
> * These persons should not receive mRNA COVID-19 vaccination at this time unless they have been evaluated by an allergist-immunologist and it is determined that the person can safely receive the vaccine (e.g., under observation, in a setting with advanced medical care available). See Appendix B for more information on ingredients included in mRNA COVID-19 vaccines.

Reasons to Question the Covid-19 Vaccination Narrative

Gary Null PhD[69]
Progressive Radio Network, January 21, 2021

---

[69] Dr. Gary Null https://vaccinenation.net/reasons-to-question-the-covid-19-vaccination-narrative/

FRAUDULENT DEATH TOLLS AS A TOOL FOR SUPPORTING THE FEAR APPEAL

Inflated Covid Cases and Fatalities Discussion Between Dr. Henele & Dr. Mercola [70]

Dr. Joseph Mercola:

In the year 2020 a death reporting policy change was instituted for the corona virus that was never applied to any other cause of death previously. The new directive said that a death is to be logged as a corona virus death even if there is no proof but there is a suspicion that a person's death was corona virus. Doctors could use a person coughing, just once, as evidence of coronavirus. This meant that people with co-morbid conditions such as diabetes, heart failure, etc., who were already moribund, would be logged as corona virus deaths even if there is no proof that coronavirus had anything to do with the actual deaths. This policy change was applied just before the corona virus started to affect the US population, and only applied to corona virus and no other diseases. Along with that policy change, there was an incentive given to health professionals and hospitals, for each new coronavirus patient they log, as it was announced that additional funds would be available to those hospitals for each corona virus patient they register. In the for-profit medical system, such policies would insure the inflation of supposed corona virus death numbers and the funds would act as incentives if not outright coercion to inflate the numbers.

A New York Post article reported on a CDC report about the conditions under which the people that "supposedly" died, due to the corona virus, should be accounted for. In the year 2020, the CDC itself said that their own number of the coronavirus deaths, that they had reported, and that the media was using to tell the population, was wrong. They said, at that time, that actually, 94% of the people that died had an average of 2.6 comorbid conditions (in the year 2021 the figure was revised to 3.8 co-morbid conditions[71]). This means that the people who were dying were not randomly anyone in the population but rather specifically those with

---

[70] https://play.acast.com/s/take-control-of-your-health-with-dr-mercola/900c752f-9b1b-4917-89de-c727bd95fc72
[71] www.drbvip.com

compromised immune systems due to being afflicted by co-morbid conditions such as diabetes, high blood pressure, cancer, obesity, etc. So they did not die <u>FROM</u> corona virus but only <u>WITH</u> corona virus – and that is considering that a fraudulent test was used to determine that they supposedly had corona virus in their bodies at the time of death or the corona virus was said to be the cause of death, on the death certificate, out of suspicion without proof.

Final, Irrefutable Proof that the Covid-19 Pandemic Never Existed[72]

- Dr. Vernon Coleman

Therefore, this means that, according to the CDC itself, only 6% of the reported deaths were "supposedly" (still unproven) due to the corona virus alone. This also would mean that there was, at that time, proof that the corona virus was neither deadly to "everyone" nor as deadly as the supposed numbers were appearing to be or were being promoted as. <u>This means that, in fact, there was not, at that time, and never was previously a corona virus "pandemic."</u>[73] Instead, there was only a fraudulent "testing pandemic" caused by the purposeful wrong use of an inappropriate test which was known to produce false positives, especially in the way it was purposely being used (with high number [30-40] of cycle thresholds). So, if the advertised number of corona virus deaths is being promoted in the media as 500,000 then the real number according to the CDC was only 30,000. Yet the media has continued to promote the higher number without being corrected by the government or health officials.

94% of Americans who died from COVID-19 had contributing conditions: CDC

August 31, 2020[74]

Ninety-four percent of Americans who died from COVID-19 had other "types of health conditions and contributing causes" in addition to the virus, according to a new CDC report.

---

[72] **FINAL, IRREFUTABLE PROOF THAT THE COVID-19 PANDEMIC NEVER EXISTED**
https://brandnewtube.com/watch/final-irrefutable-proof-that-the-covid-19-pandemic-never-existed_JmPw8cUxQG1w7NP.html
[73] IBID
[74] https://nypost.com/2020/08/31/94-of-americans-who-died-from-covid-19-had-contributing-conditions/

As of Monday, the US has surpassed 6 million coronavirus cases and 183,000 deaths, Johns Hopkins University statistics show.

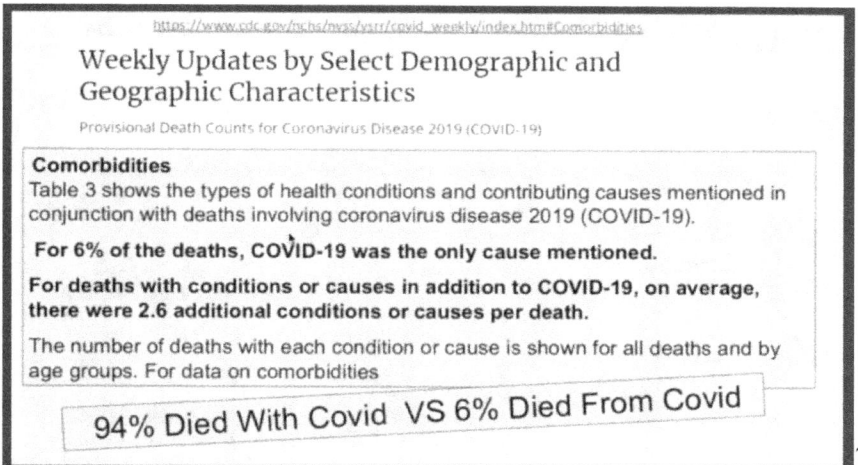

However, as of Monday, August 24, 2020 the death total was being reported as 183,000. So in reality, at that time, only 10,980 could be said to have died from the corona virus alone. The same reporting of the higher number as the deaths from coronavirus, continues as of the time of this writing (May 2021). We may then correctly ask why would the CDC continue to allow everyone to think that all people are equally susceptible to die from corona virus disease and why was the high incorrect number of deaths, used by the media, not corrected by them? Additionally, why would the media, which has the capacity to do fact checking on their own, continue to report the higher number as the "death toll" from the corona virus disease instead of correcting the error and reporting the correct reduced number? The answer, of course, is collusion and corruption at the CDC and in the news media for ulterior motives. These issues coupled with the also admitted fraudulent conflation of deaths from corona virus with deaths from all causes, including car accidents, the FLU, and or pneumonia with the total supposed corona virus deaths means that the actual death total was much lower still.

---

[75] https://www.drbvip.com/courses/new-uncensored-content-video-resource-library-archive/567775-in-the-know-with-dr-b-video-archive-feb-2021/1946732-pandemic-predictions-and-actual-deaths-wef-in-the-know-with-dr-b-full-video-mp4

Birx says government is classifying all deaths of patients with coronavirus as 'COVID-19' deaths, regardless of cause[76]

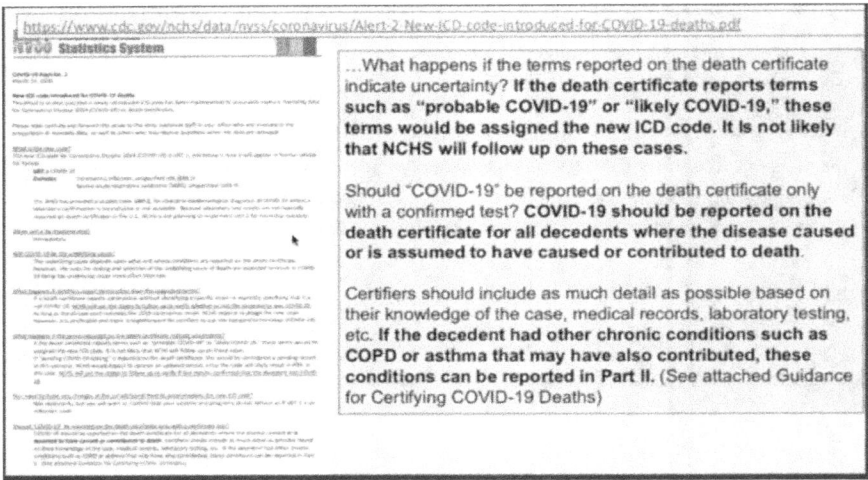

CDC director acknowledges hospitals have a monetary incentive to overcount coronavirus deaths[77]

| August 01, 2020

---

[76] https://www.foxnews.com/politics/birx-says-government-is-classifying-all-deaths-of-patients-with-coronavirus-as-covid-19-deaths-regardless-of-cause
[77] https://www.washingtonexaminer.com/news/cdc-director-acknowledges-hospitals-have-a-monetary-incentive-to-overcount-coronavirus-deaths

IMPLICATIONS SO FAR

The manner of the recording of the deaths, supposedly due to corona virus, and allowing that to be presented by politicians and in the media as a large number of deaths that can strike "anyone" down irrespective of their health condition, their comorbid conditions, the condition of their immune system are signs of corruption and collusion. Adding to that, the factors of not presenting known safe and effective methods to promote prevention and healing such as supplements, and safe drugs, the purposeful discouraging of such information by suppressing its dissemination, fraudulently disparaging the alternative treatments and encouraging media corporations to censor/cancel anyone talking about such prevention and curative measures, demonstrates a case against the politicians, scientists, the health agencies and the media, that is involved, for reckless endangerment and disregard for human life, depraved indifference and crimes against humanity.

CHANGE IN HOW CYCLE THRESHOLDS ARE MANIPULATED IN THE PCR TESTS TO PRODUCE THE DESIRED NUMBER OF "CASES" SUFFICIENT TO SCARE THE POPULATION AND JUSTIFY MEDICAL TYRANNY

In early 2020 the PCR test was instituted to determine how many people were supposedly in a diseased state due to the corona virus. Firstly, according to the scientist creator of the PCR test, PCR test is not to be used as a diagnostic test for any disease. Secondly, even if a person has the virus that does not mean that have any disease, let alone a disease caused by the virus. Therefore, calling people who may have the virus as a "case" like someone sick in a hospital, was disingenuous at best and purposely criminally fraudulent as evidenced by the continued use of that wrong criteria to scare the population. Using the known wrong test and classifications, the "cases of covid-19 coronavirus" jumped due to the change in testing and counting method from what it had been previously.[78] This caused apparently surging numbers of people supposedly infected, sick, and dying of covid-19 disease throughout the year. There were many complaints about this issue, from scientists and others, throughout the year, yet the WHO and CDC continued implementing this metric worldwide and

---

[78] https://www.forbes.com/sites/brucelee/2020/02/13/new-coronavirus-covid-19-counting-method-leads-to-jump-in-cases-deaths/?sh=5435ea8316af

the result, as expected, was large numbers of supposed "cases" that was used to scare the population into using masks, social distancing, and lockdowns. Thus, the manufactured false support, for belief in a supposed pandemic and the implementation of draconian political actions, was in place. Then after months of complaints to CDC, by some conscientious scientists and others, at the beginning of the year, 2021 changes were finally made to the method of determining so-called "cases" that turns out to be a politically and economically advantageous time for the democratic party, the WHO and CDC.

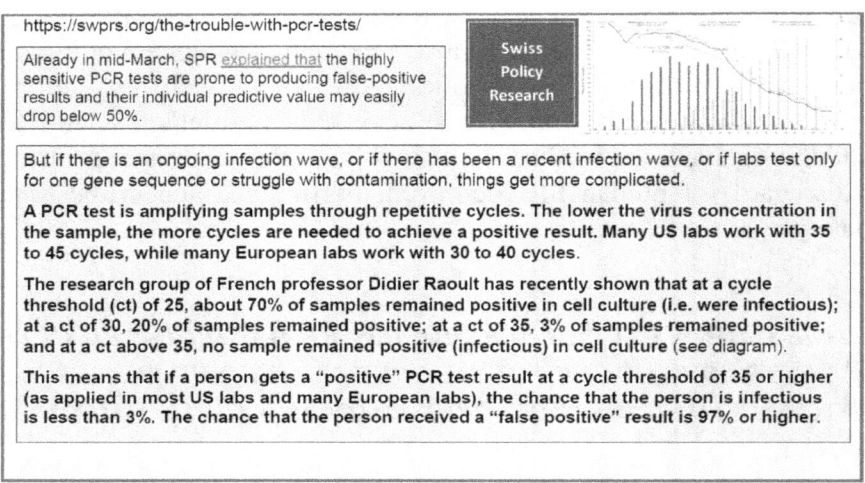

Most people are not aware that on January 20, 2021, the same day as the inauguration of the new president of the USA, the World Health Organization lowered the cycle threshold to be used in determining who supposedly is a covid 19 "case". Since the cycle threshold determines how many people will show as "positive" (which actually has no meaning in terms of showing who is actually sick or who can become sick and/or infect others), this means that there will be definitely fewer people appearing as infected cases of covid 19. This occurred after months, at least since summer 2020, of complaints by some ethical scientists and others, that firstly, the PCR tests are inappropriate to determine who is infected and who has the covid 19 disease and so, even the inventor of the PCR, Kary Mullis, said it should not be used at all for determining any infection. Additionally, the complaint is that the cycle thresholds are too high which means there will be as many as 90% false positives. The FDA (Food and Drug Administration) apparently agreed with Dr. Kary Mullis, yet the same testing protocol continued to be used, that is, until January 2021. The Swedish Public Health agency has determined that PCR tests cannot be used to diagnose covid 19 disease and who is contagious; why has their scientific finding and conclusion not been disseminated around the world? Answer: to continue the fraud of using PCR testing to scare the population and make everyone think they are infected and diseased and then accept experimental vaccines.

SWEDEN SAYS PCR TESTS "CANNOT BE USED TO DETERMINE WHETHER SOMEONE IS CONTAGIOUS"

By Arjun Walia – May 21, 2021

WHO lowers PCR cycle count, causing less positives on the day Biden becomes President[79]

January 20, 2021

One hour after Biden inaugurated, WHO changes COVID testing criteria[80]

COVID cases plummet after WHO changes testing protocol on Biden's Inauguration Day[81]

02/8/2021

---

[79] https://thecoloradoherald.com/2021/who-lowers-pcr-cycle-count-causing-less-positives-on-the-day-biden-becomes-president/
[80] https://www.lifesitenews.com/news/one-hour-after-biden-inaugurated-who-changes-covid-testing-criteria
https://www.who.int/news/item/20-01-2021-who-information-notice-for-ivd-users-2020-05
[81] https://www.lifesitenews.com/news/covid-cases-plummet-after-who-changes-testing-protocol-on-bidens-inauguration-day

WHO says COVID-19 deaths plunged by 20 percent last week[82]

New cases are also showcasing steady declines across the world. *Feb. 23, 2021*

REFLECTIONS

So, on the fraudulent basis of the PCR test, the WHO and the CDC, along with the politicians and the media, manufactured a "pandemic" that never was, from the beginning and continued using fraudulent death count numbers to maintain the fraud. But now, since president Trump is officially out of the office and president Biden is in, now the CDC and WHO have decided that the scare pressure of the "covid disease" can be lowered (from 40 cycles to 28 cycles)[83]. This reduction allows a planned reduced cause to scare the population and gives cover to reduce the mask-wearing by vaccinated persons, reduce social distancing and lockdowns and allow the economy to recover giving credit to the new governing democratic party regime. Additionally, with the lowered cycle PCR tests, since the dangerous and unproven so-called "vaccines" have been introduced and are being administered (since December 2020), now it would be possible to claim that those getting the vaccines are not being infected with coronavirus and also show less so-called "covid cases" and attribute the reduction to the vaccines[84] instead of to natural herd immunity and the use of supplements and known effective drugs.[85] The findings by Canadian doctors and others, around the world, reveals that the disease referred to as "coronavirus or "covid 19" should not be a motive for undue concern or fear as there are supplements and drugs to prevent and cure the disease and there is no concern of children catching or spreading or asymptomatic spreading; so school closings and lockdowns are not necessary.[86]

---

[82] https://thehill.com/changing-america/well-being/medical-advances/540245-who-says-covid-19-deaths-plunged-by-20-percent
[83] https://prn.fm/gary-null-show-05-07-21/
[84] ibid
[85] CANADIAN DOCTORS SPEAK OUT ON COVID
https://canadianpatriot.org/2021/04/27/canadian-doctors-speak-out-on-covid/
[86] https://youtu.be/UVzxu5Uxd10

Asymptomatic spreading of covid 19 is *"de minimis"* and "covid 19 recovered patients have not significant risk of recurrence…none..none…they get natural immunity".[87]

By ignoring the findings of qualified health personnel and continuing to use the subterfuge of the reduced cycle tests and the media fearmongering, the politicians and supposed health "authorities" could continue to encourage/deceive people into getting vaccinated and by doing so remaining under the control of government and possibly becoming debilitated, sick and registered in the government systems as docketed persons who have received the unknown substance that can be part of future manipulations including lowered fertility and reduced life expectancy. Such is the corruption and collusion between the politicians, the media, the pharmaceutical industry, the CDC, and the World Health Organization, the latter two supposedly dedicated to promoting world health. A possible glitch in the coronavirus PCR test and the pseudo-vaccine deception is that many of those who have been vaccinated have later tested positive for coronavirus, AFTER BEING VACCINATED, (so-called breakthrough cases –many of which are being hidden from the public[88]) even at the reduced PCR cycle level. This means that either the vaccines do not work and are allowing peoples immune systems to be infected or that the vaccine itself is causing the infections. In any case it is wise to avoid falling into the delusions and confidence schemes of the government officials and supposed health "authorities" who have, in reality, revealed themselves as craven, duplicitous, corrupt, rapacious sociopaths.[89]

---

[87] Dr. Peter McCullough [covid 19 update. https://youtu.be/UVzxu5Uxd10]
[88] https://youtu.be/UVzxu5Uxd10
https://breggin.com/
[89] ibid

MORE EXAMPLES OF THE CORRUPTIONS REVEALED IN THE YEAR 2020

The year 2020 also revealed how certain wealthy corporations, especially those leading the technocracy, the "Big Tech" and social media companies, and their owners, such as Jeff Bezos and Elon Musk, profited by the lockdowns that caused millions of businesses to go into bankruptcy and close for good.

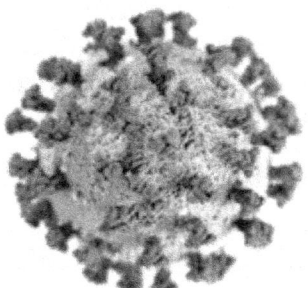

Above: the widely distributed and **not proven** artist rendition of the **theoretical appearance** of the supposed corona virus that supposedly causes covid 19 disease.

The year 2020 revealed the compromised and corrupt state of the mainstream media and social media companies as they engaged in open propaganda and censorship of any dissenting views such as those calling out the false and contradictory information that was and still is being put out by the government agencies, the CDC, the WHO, and the media about the nature of coronavirus infection, disease and treatments. One such deception is the visual representation of a theoretical virus that has never been seen (isolated) from the body since an alternative virology theory is that viruses are "exosomes" excreted by the body itself, due to disease, for varied reasons, including poor diet, environmental poisons like factory and auto pollution, geoengineering weather modification chemicals from airplanes, toxic thoughts, relationships, and stress. Therefore, the so-called "virus" could be the result of and not the cause of infection and disease, due to a lowered immune system. This would mean that trying to make a vaccine to stop the wrong cause of disease (the virus) would never stop the disease. This direction of science would be following the apparently failed model of "germ theory" of disease that claims disease occurs due to germs or viruses and neglects the concept put forward by "terrain theory", the idea that lowered immunity *allows* the diseases and pathogens, from within the body and from outside the body, to attack the body and cause disease.[90] In this context, perhaps a better way to think of disease processes is integrally, meaning that the terrain or health condition of a body is susceptible to pathogens (germs and virus) deleterious effects by being out of a healthy state. This concept follows the Ancient Egyptian idea of disease called "ukhedu." Therefore, the terrain and germ theories can be thought of, not as being mutually exclusive, but rather as being interrelated. The health of the terrain is the most important. Then controlling exposure to viruses and bacteria from outside the body (including man-made) and controlling the development of potential pathogens from the viruses and bacteria that reside in the body and not allowing them to come out of their natural balance, and become pathogenic, is important.

Twitter Isn't Censoring Accounts to Keep Users 'Safe', It Is Using Its Power to Spoon-feed the World Establishment Narratives
By Eva Bartlett
Global Research, May 03, 2021

The mainstream media and social media companies actively and openly censored (in 2020) and continue to censor anyone, not in line with the politicians, corporations, and supposed health agencies that stood and still stand to benefit from producing pseudo-vaccines instead of telling everyone about safe and effective vitamin and mineral supplements and proven drug therapies such as hydroxychloroquine and ivermectin to prevent and or remedy the disease that was attributed to a virus, the existence of which up to now (May 2021) no proof of its full genetic sequence has been presented[91]. Therefore, the idea that there is something called "corona virus" that causes "corona virus or covid 19 disease" is not proven since the isolated genetic sequence of such a virus has not been isolated and presented. Hence, this is only a hypothesis and not

---

[90] https://www.westonaprice.org/health-topics/notes-from-yesteryear/germ-theory-versus-terrain-the-wrong-side-won-the-day/
Dr. Sam Bailey 2020 The Year Medicine Lost Contact
https://www.youtube.com/watch?v=qP8bfJG7dQw
https://www.knowingthetruth.com/exosomes-vs-viruses-scientific-theories-explained/
[91] https://redpilluniversity.org/2021/02/14/chinas-chief-epidemiologist-admits-covid-19-was-never-proven-to-exist/

a fact that has been proven; therefore, it is only an assumption, not a proven fact. Furthermore, this means that any so-called vaccine based on whatever the genetic "snippets" (pieces, fragments of what they believe is a virus causing disease) that have been thought to be part of such a theoretical (not proven) virus cannot be effective against any given disease, since there is not even proof that the genetic fragment that is being used in an inappropriate test for the supposed "corona virus disease" has not been proven to be part of any theoretical (not proven) virus, let alone the theoretical/hypothesized virus theoretically hypothesized to be the cause of the disease that has been observed in elderly populations and people with co-morbid health conditions. The presence of the supposed virus, based on the hypothetical and thin scientific evidence used to create a test for it is so wanting that the tests have such numbers of false positives that the test itself is useless. Nevertheless, it continues to be used, despite these well-known facts. Thus, the scientific community is in the dark about whether or not the disease is caused by a virus, yet there has been a scientific race to claim to have proven it as a fact in order to reap the rewards of scientific discovery and financial remuneration related to more faulty testing and experimental theoretical therapies. Politicians have latched onto the supposed proofs presented by the fraudulent scientists and modelers to use those as an excuse to call the situation a "pandemic" and use that as a basis for imposing "emergency policies" which amount to medical martial law and police state tyranny.

Tanzania Kicks Out WHO After Goat and Papaya Samples Came COVID-19 Positive
-GreatGameIndia May 11, 2020

Finally, the reference to the disease that started affecting some people in the year 2020, referred to as "sars covid 2" as if it is related to the previous disease that was named "*SARS*" is also theoretical since the previous "sars" was also not isolated and its genetic sequence was never proven either. The comparison between the supposed fragments of each sample, being incomplete and therefore, its original source not fully known, means that the comparison itself is like comparing two things, neither of which its origin is known and having only parts of each and then saying that some part of those matches so they are related. Therefore, the association between the two supposed viruses is a hypothesis, based on theories, at best and corrupt speculation, based on greed and competition, at worst, supported by politicians and their propaganda and the mainstream media echo chambers supporting the supposed scientific findings that were never proven in the first place, while going forward and focusing everyone's attention on the disease and apparent soaring infection rates based on fraudulent use of an inappropriate test for a virus that has not even been proven to exist.

DEMOCRAT PARTY VS. REPUBLICAN PARTY POLITICS IN THE RESPONSE TO CORONA VIRUS DISEASE (COVID 19)

The **year 2020 revealed** the extent that especially the democratic party governors would go to support the lockdowns and misuse of supposed emergency powers to make the lockdowns more severe than the states governed by republican governors. Some speculated that this was done to cause economic failure, using the virus as an excuse, so as to cause discontent that would lead to the loss by republican party president Donald Trump, of the presidency in the elections held in November 2020. Yet, the lockdowns were imposed worldwide on healthy individuals, something never done before in human history, and they were continued after the election. Thus, the indication is that the agenda behind the masking and lockdowns goes beyond the politics of a single country but involves the politics and economics worldwide, the overpowering the world democratic and non-democratic governing systems and economies.

Early on, in the supposed "pandemic" the UK government assessed that corona virus was no worse than the annual FLU but nevertheless continued to follow the dictates of the WHO, thereby proving that even though the UK separated from the European Union, they were still bound by another system of control, the medical martial law of a WHO treaty that forces the signatories to follow the WHO dictates. Therefore, being a member of the WHO signs away the individual rights of the signatory countries. That means that whoever controls the WHO (including potential criminals and sociopaths) can impose medical martial law and medical tyranny on any of the member countries (overriding their national laws or national sovereignty) or by coercion any other country that needs to deal with a signatory country, potentially giving them world-wide control and power to impose policies that can lead to corrupt medical advice to benefit pharmaceutical companies, up to and including population reduction agendas of the power elites.

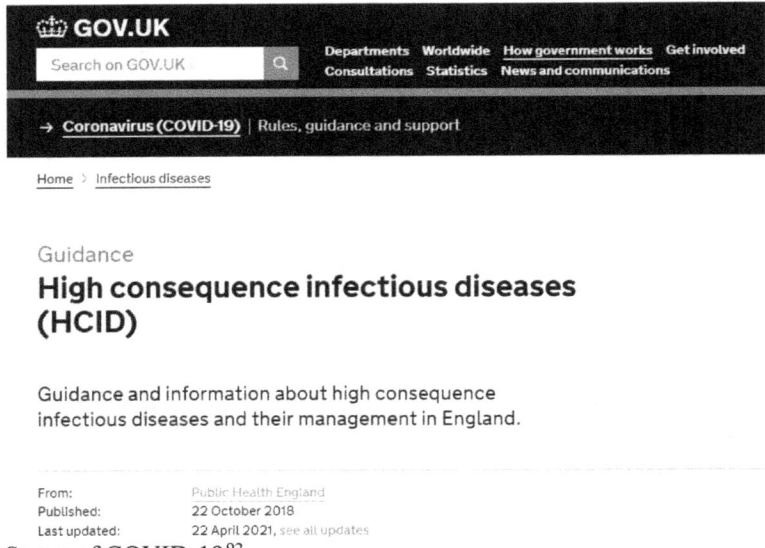

Status of COVID-19[92]

As of 19 March 2020, COVID-19 is no longer considered to be a high consequence infectious disease (HCID) in the UK. There are many diseases which can cause serious illness which are not classified as HCIDs.
The Advisory Committee on Dangerous Pathogens (ACDP) is also of the opinion that COVID-19 should no longer be classified as an HCID. The World Health Organization (WHO) continues to consider COVID-19 as a Public Health Emergency of International Concern (PHEIC), therefore the need to have a national, coordinated response remains and this is being met by the government's COVID-19 response.

The year 2020 revealed how willingly people would be to turn on each other, out of fear and or ignorance, those willing to comply with authority figures, with the help of the media, calling those who did not want to comply, "Covidiots" or "covid deniers" and ridiculing them for saying that the virus was no worse than a regular FLU[93] season and or that presidents and governors have no right to impose such medical tyranny policies. By the end of the year 2020 it became evident that the countries and states that did not impose mask-wearing, social distancing, and lockdowns had no different outcomes or had better outcomes than the states and countries that

---

[92] https://www.gov.uk/guidance/high-consequence-infectious-diseases-hcid
[93] HTTPS://BRANDNEWTUBE.COM/WATCH/FINAL-IRREFUTABLE-PROOF-THAT-THE-COVID-19-PANDEMIC-NEVER-EXISTED_JMPW8CUXQG1W7NP.HTML

did impose those policies. Also, it was revealed that the year 2020 apparently did not have excess mortality, more people dying than in usual years, supposedly because of the virus. Neither of these findings have been widely disseminated to the public, which continues to believe there was widespread death that continues to this day, due to the supposed pandemic. In early 2021 it was discovered that the FLU cases plummeted from the previous year, from 38,000,000 in season 2019-202 to only 1,822 in the 2020-2021 FLU season. Clearly, the FLU cases have been conflated with or simply reclassified as covid 19 cases.

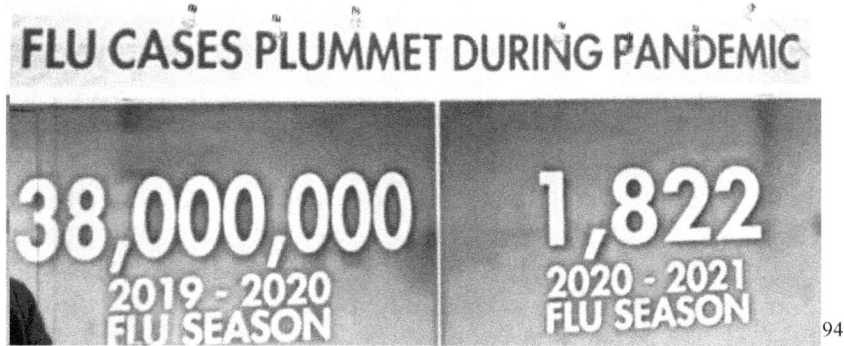

[94]

All the final numbers for the total deaths for 2020 will not be in for some time, but so far the indication is an average year as previous years. If this is confirmed it means that the so-called COVID/coronavirus impact was not what the public was made to fear, based on the estimates given by the government health officials and politicians. Additionally, as of now, it is possible to say that the impact of corona virus disease was indeed no worse than the regular FLU.[95] Actually, the finding so far is that children were more at risk from the FLU than the corona virus since the FLU actually kills children while there are almost no deaths at all among the younger population that can be attributable to corona virus disease (covid 19). So, indeed the FLU was and remains more dangerous to the whole population, since it also sickens and kills many children, than the corona virus ever did, since the corona virus disease has almost no effect, at all, on children. Therefore, the corona virus has definitely proved more dangerous to the older populations, particularly those with co-morbid conditions, but not dangerous to children or healthy adults. The conclusion that whatever the disease, first referred to as "Wuhan virus" and now referred to as corona "virus" or "covid 19", was not deadly to all people was already known since the time when northern Italy was first affected and also of the Diamond

---

[94] https://www.drbvip.com/
[95] ibid

Princes cruise where only some elderly passengers were affected; this same finding was known at least since late spring (April 2020) when it was obvious that the elderly with co-morbid conditions were the susceptible population, but the official policies did not and have not yet changed to conform to the real "scientific" findings. This conclusion was reached by the UK government as early as 19 March 2020, yet there was a decision to comply with the dictates of the WHO which continued to treat the disease as if it was a true "Public Health Emergency of International Concern (PHEIC)". Here is the PROOF (document image above) that covid-19 was downgraded by the UK government in March 2020.

Thus, it was known early on that covid 19 was not a serious disease necessitating the designation as a pandemic. It was also known that it was the older persons with comorbid conditions (diabetes, high blood pressure, heart disease, etc.) are really the susceptible population, though the media and the supposed health agencies, NIAID (headed by Anthony Fauci), NIH, CDC, etc. ignored those findings and continued pushing fear among all populations regardless of age or health levels. They continued pushing for more general mask-wearing, school closings, social distancing, and lockdowns along with waiting for experimental and dangerous drugs and vaccines and discouraging taking any known medicines or supplements to bolster the immune system, which, again, are known to be safe and effective for preventing infection and reducing mortality from the so-called corona virus disease (covid 19).

THE FALLACY OF EXCESS MORTALITY DUE TO CORONA VIRUS

Johns Hopkins: COVID Has Had No Effect On US Death Rate[96]

November 26, 2020

An argument used to support the fear-mongering about the corona virus and the need for masks, social distancing and lockdowns is the supposed excess deaths that the virus was supposed to have caused. Excess deaths are inordinate extra deaths caused by an unusual cause. In other words, "excess deaths" are deaths that occur "in addition to" the regular or average number of deaths that occur each year. As of the findings of researches like the one undertaken by Johns Hopkins, the indications are that there were no inordinate numbers of deaths

---

[96] https://www.libertariannews.org/2020/11/26/study-covid-has-had-no-effect-on-us-death-rate/

considering the growing population and the increasing numbers of aged individuals in the population; though this knowledge has also had little effect in changing the policies of the people in government, health officials or the mainstream media messages.

A closer look at U.S. deaths due to COVID-19[97]

November 22, 2020

COVIDIOCY OR COVIDMANIA

In early 2020, there was remarkable rapidity of the general population's willingness to accept the dictates of supposed health and political leaders to adopt fear and callout others who did not agree with the officials and then acted out of consuming fear by immediately adopting mask-wearing, social distancing, and lockdowns and calling them "Covidiots" or "covid denier" or "conspiracy theorists". Now it is clear that the rapidity of the general population's compliance with the dictates of supposed authority figures and their continued compliance with their dictates, allegedly based on advice from medical experts, who in most instances were found to be either compromised, fraudulent or wrong in their projections, predictions and therapies may be referred to as "covidmania." Covidmania may be thought of as an expression of cult behavior. People generally have been degraded to such a degree as to see the politicians and health officials as unquestioned leaders leading to the greater good for all and anyone questioning that is an enemy; this is the delusion of a cult mind.[98] So the people calling others "Covidiots for not accepting the government policies are the actual "Covidiots" suffering from "covidmania". Covidmania or "virus mania" may be viewed as a situation wherein people have become so ignorant, deluded, and stressed with fear and confusion that they will readily accept irrational, illogical, ineffectual, erroneous, or even dangerous dictates and impositions by people who have arrogated for themselves the right to impose such policies on the population. Those dictates and policies or powers are not in the country's constitution or any law that has been ratified by any electoral process in which people

---

[97] https://web.archive.org/web/20201126043553/https://www.jhunewsletter.com/article/2020/11/a-closer-look-at-u-s-deaths-due-to-covid-19
[98] https://www.bitchute.com/video/cWCE1h0ZMk4g/
https://www.bitchute.com/video/rTPzMkTAxQOH/

have given those right with their informed consent. So, those who were, at the outset, calling others "covidiots", for initially refusing to wear masks and accept lockdowns out of ignorance or legitimate concern about what the authorities were saying, were the ones suffering "covidmania" or "virus mania"[99] due to their degraded state of mind owing to a degraded state of life and degraded sense of personal sovereignty and dysfunctional ego-personality that was in need of having others make decisions for them (i.e. a cult mentality).

Virus Mania: How the Medical Industry Continually Invents Epidemics, Making Billion Dollar Profits at Our Expense
–January 28, 2021[100]

A Book Review of Virus Mania: How the Medical Industry Continually Invents Epidemics, Making Billion-Dollar Profits at Our Expense[101]

By Etienne de Harven, MD. May 9, 2020

---

[99] VIRUS MANIA: CORONA/COVID-19, MEASLES, SWINE FLU, CERVICAL CANCER, AVIAN FLU, SARS, BSE, HEPATITIS C, AIDS, POLIO, SPANISH FLU. HOW THE MEDICAL ... MAKING BILLION-DOLLAR PROFITS AT OUR EXPENSE PAPERBACK – JANUARY 28, 2021
[100] ibid
[101] https://www.lewrockwell.com/2020/05/no_author/a-book-review-of-virus-mania-how-the-medical-industry-continually-invents-epidemics-making-billion-dollar-profits-at-our-expense/

THE CORRUPTION OF THE CDC AND THE DUBIOUS CORONA VIRUS SO-CALLED VACCINES

Researcher David Martin, a professor, and patent expert seems to have uncovered evidence that the CDC (Centers for Disease Control and prominent billionaires (members of the worldwide power elites) conspired in reference to patenting the COVID/Coronavirus illegally.[102] Additionally, he also holds that there is evidence of a conspiracy to produce a more virulent pathogen and then to commit acts of terror using the media and "hype" to attract investors seeking profit. Dr. Gary Null, and many other scientists and health researchers, have researched and found supplements and drugs that act as safe methods to prevent or heal from coronavirus infection; so why are these scientifically proven remedies ignored or denied by the power elite and their technocratic managers (the politicians and the managers of corporations and the media as well as their employees- including health officials)? For the answer we may consider: greed, delusion, hunger for power, hubris and sociopathy.

Subsequent documentation has supported the findings of David Martin as well as revelations of information hidden by the Chinese government.

Gravitas: The interview China tried to hide | Wuhan Coronavirus | Dr. Ai Fen[103]
•Apr 3, 2020

===============

Natural Love In The Time Of Covid [104/105]

---

[102] https://www.davidmartin.world/wp-content/uploads/2021/01/The_Fauci_COVID-19_Dossier.pdf
https://prn.fm/gary-null-show-01-22-21/
https://prn.fm/gary-null-show-01-21-21/
https://prn.fm/gary-null-show-01-18-21/
[103] https://youtu.be/beDmuDDknNI
[104] https://vaccinenation.net/natural-love-in-the-time-of-covid/
[105] https://vaccinenation.net/reasons-to-question-the-covid-19-vaccination-narrative/

TRENDS JOURNAL TRENDS IN GETTING HEALTHY February 9, 2021

My producer and I have scoured the peer-reviewed literature on the National Institutes of Health's Library of Medicine database to identify compelling studies that may warrant vitamin, antioxidant, and botanical supplementation as a means to protect ourselves from coronavirus and other viral infections. These have been shown to either have strong antiviral properties in general or have known bimolecular effects to strengthen the immune system against microbial infection.

Self-Delusion, Disempowerment, Spiritual bankruptcy and Political Enslavement

Maat Philosophy is first and foremost about "truth" and "righteousness" based on truth. There are two forms of truth or ethics, the truth of the secular and the truth of the non-secular. In this volume we are approaching the issues of fascism, police state and medical tyranny from the perspective of secular ethics wisdom of Maat. However, it should be known that the secular truth is founded in the spiritual truth of the all-encompassing and universal nature of humanity and Creation. The Ancient Egyptian wisdom of Maat holds that a population that is not able to or is not willing to live by truth will compose a society of deluded individuals and their leaders will be from the ranks of kakistocracy.

A deluded society, one that is not able or is not willing to understand and follow truth is a society that devolves to tyranny and barbarism. In western society and the country USA, in particular, along with the countries that have been affected by the politics and economics of those countries (western society and the country USA), there are four forms of important untruths that are projected by the ruling class and held on to by the lower classes, which poison the society. The untruths in question have a corrosive effect on individual human cognition and conscience which corrupts politics, human interaction and economics, leading to social conflict, political polarization, rapacious corrupt economics and a culture of hate and death instead of cooperation and best practices and life. These untruths include: race and racism, terror vs. humanitarianism, democracy vs. fascism, and capitalism vs. equal opportunity. When untruth is the foundation of life then the mental capacity of the members of a society devolves to life based on delusions that hurt the deluded person and can be manipulated and exploited for unrighteous purposes. In these cases, the delusions involve a denial of truth and adherence to perspectives that sustain the social delusions, knowingly or unknowingly, that allow them to feel better about themselves and or maintain their positions in the social class of the society.

THE DELUSION (INCAPACITY AND OR UNWILLINGNESS TO FACE THE TRUTH OF) OF RACE AND RACISM.

The delusion about and belief in the concept of "race" is founded in the ignorance about the nature of humanity. There is only one "race", the "human race" and there are no individual or different races of human beings. Such a belief while being irrational because it is false is also a pathway to degraded feelings and thoughts that lead to degraded emotions and actions. In the deluded society, the belief in race and the belief in the existence of "different" races of humans that is supposedly supported by real science, to support the belief, such as genetics, is a monumental fallacy. <u>There are no races of humans; there is only one human race composed of varied ethnic and cultural groups with some individuals, in the groups, possessing surface variations in hue and physical features due to living in geographically varied climates.</u> Therefore, the belief in "race" as a "real" differentiating factor, justifying segregation and as a factor that causes one group of humans to be different from another, itself is a racist concept that acts as the foundation for delusions of superiority and inferiority as well as a basis for unscrupulous or outright sociopathic individuals or groups to manipulate people with those beliefs through demagoguery and charlatanism aimed at fomenting human divisions and conflict so as to direct the course of society to their own (demagogues and charlatans) ends and benefit.

The year 2020 revealed a continuing seething racial issue in USA culture due to the continuing support, by politicians and narcissistic personalities like Donald Trump as well as key government authorities and power elites, of institutional racism and incapacity or unwillingness to face the atrocities of the past and present, make amends, work towards correcting the causes of racial discrimination and redress past wrongs done to those previously and continuingly being discriminated, held back and or enslaved. The heinous murder by the government trained and sanctioned police, of George Floyd, sparked unprecedented protests in the USA and around the world, over racial injustice and in particular, the police brutality visited on the lower classes of society but especially the poor, the middle class, and the African American and Latino members of the population. After his death, unprecedented protests against police brutality, especially toward black people, quickly spread across the United States and internationally. Yet, though there may have been a temporary reduction in "racial" police killings, as of early 2021 no concrete changes in the institutional, social, policing, or legal systems have occurred, just as no major changes occur after mass shootings, even those involving children. The point is that changes in these areas have not, in the past, been desired, by the power elites who control government, presumably as a method of allowing violent situations in society that are ripe for promoting fear among the lower classes along with legitimizing militarization of the police.

THE DELUSION (INCAPACITY AND OR UNWILLINGNESS TO FACE THE TRUTH OF) OF TERRORIST VS. THE GOOD GUY.

The country USA is replete with examples of successful false flag, psychological disinformation operations, and propaganda efforts that cause USA citizens to believe that their government and their country are the "good guys" while other countries are wrong or stupid or bad, outlaw, etc. The belief in oneself or one's country as the "good guy" is preferable to the realization that one's country is, in fact, the foremost purveyor of international and national terrorism in the year 2021 as it was in the time of Martin Luther King.

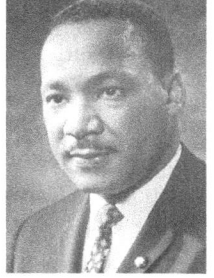

As I have walked among the desperate, rejected, and angry young men, I have told them that Molotov cocktails and rifles would not solve their problems. I have tried to offer them my deepest compassion while maintaining my conviction that social change comes most meaningfully through nonviolent action. But they asked, and rightly so, "What about Vietnam?" They asked if our own nation wasn't using massive doses of violence to solve its problems, to bring about the changes it wanted. Their questions hit home, and I knew that I could never again raise my voice against the violence of the oppressed in the ghettos without having first spoken clearly to the greatest purveyor of violence in the world today: my own government. For the sake of those boys, for the sake of this government, for the sake of the hundreds of thousands trembling under our violence, I cannot be silent.
                                                        -Martin Luther King Jr.[106]

During the George W. Bush presidency a major lie was that the country "Iraq has weapons of mass destruction" that they intend to use on the USA. This lie was perpetrated by the president, his staff, the spy agencies, and the media. It led to hundreds of thousands of deaths and lives destroyed and no one suffered any consequences. The same thing

---

[106] "BEYOND VIETNAM"
Author: King, Martin Luther, Jr. Date: April 4, 1967

occurred under the presidency of Barak Obama in reference to multiple drone killings that included women and children. Additionally, Obama, Joe Biden, and Hillary Clinton were principally responsible for the war on the country Syria and the country Libya, which was destroyed. The lies and law-breaking were justified in the media and by congress, people, ignored or were later portrayed as "errors" or "misguided" and not wrong or corrupt but legitimate, efforts to "keep America safe" (another three-word meme propaganda phrase).

Like being racist and or practicing or supporting racist social norms, but not wanting to think of oneself as a racist, the delusion of being good is often used as a support for untold wrongdoing. People want to think of their country and by extension, of themselves, as being "good" and that means that if the country does something wrong it is explained away as a mistake or actions by a few "bad apples", individuals who are stupid or corrupt. The coping thought, by the individuals in the society, is that those stupid or corrupt "individuals" are not the country; so the country is not stupid or corrupt or illegitimate or even wrong, and neither are its rulers. Thus, whatever the leaders did was an anomaly and not the norm. In this way, people can avoid looking critically or historically and realize that the supposed anomalies are endemic foundations of an ordinary policy of their country and that they are complicit in the corruption of their country's policies. Therefore they do not have to face that they are supporting the same unrighteousness, criminality, and war crimes that seem to be visited on others now but will eventually be visited on themselves by their own corrupt rulers. Even though the USA destroyed other countries and invaded or toppled the governments in over 100 countries in the last 100 years and became an empire, the justification is that the USA is good and trying to bring "democracy" around the world; as if the USA had the right to impose policies on other countries, regardless of if they were actually good or not, or as if the so-called form of government called "democracy" has proven itself as a benevolent political system instead of a barbarous imperial government.

USA democracy is actually no democracy at all and never was. It began as a republican representative government for white land owners aristocrats with a capitalist economy founded on slavery and indentured servitude; now it has developed into a sociopathic, barbarous *fascist totalitarian surveillance police-state.* Living under a willful delusion, people rationalize the thought that since the country is not bad and I am not bad, and it's only the "bad apples", therefore, that does not mean that "we" as a country are bad. With this rationalization ordinary people never face the reality that "they" all reap the rewards of the killing, raping, and pillaging of other countries (war crimes) that "their" country perpetrates and the allowance of corporations to exploit workers nationally and in other countries, steal their wealth and natural resources and then promote neo-feudalism and the totalitarian surveillance police state within the USA. This delusion allows its believers to support a false reality about their own country that supports untold suffering around the world as well as in their own country, as the corporatocracy exploits the deluded population that allows the internal and external barbarism policies, wars, and exploitations. So there is external (international) barbarism and empire and internally (domestic) there is socio-economic exploitation that can only be described as either internal (domestic) neo-colonialism or neo-feudalism and domestic fascism. In a modern context the description for USA society, politics, and economics as a *fascist totalitarian surveillance police-state* is applicable. This makes USA citizens, that support the delusion of their country as being the "good guy", complicit in their country's wrongdoing and also makes them eligible for receiving the terror repercussions of their delusion. It is their own delusion perpetrated on themselves by their own willful ignorance, greed, and lack of empathy that have allowed their own government, which is the same government that they approved of (by paying taxes and agreeing to vote for the lesser of two evil candidates that are put up by the power elites) when it perpetrated the wrongdoing, the torture, destruction, and subjugation of other countries on their behalf. This is the result of not facing the truth that the USA is the foremost terrorist country in the world and taking responsibility by taking action to stop it when it could have been stopped.

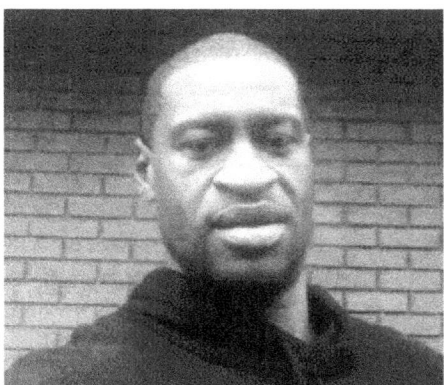

George Perry Floyd Jr. (October 14, 1973 – May 25, 2020)

George Perry Floyd Jr. was, at the time of his death, only the latest victim of thousands of police killings. His death and the death of others sparked violent protests and anger worldwide, which were not opposed by the power elite even as they sought to stop protests about the lockdowns. Instead of taking responsibility for the perpetration and maintenance of racism and redressing, making amends, seeking forgiveness, for the wrongs and harms done, the leaders continue spouting platitudes of support and unity while upholding and empowering the institutional policies as in previous times that allow police brutality and exploitation of the population. Others in the majority "white" community continued to deny they have any responsibility, saying that the wrongs were done by their ancestors and they, the descendants, are not responsible, while still others take a pathological stance claiming that all "white" people are racists simply by being white.

The foolish idea that "all white people are racists simply by being born white" is false on its face, and misses the point of institutionalized and self-perpetuating delusions in the government and corporate institutions, that foment racism and racial disparities that manifest as deluded notions about race that support unconscious institutional racism. Those delusions are exacerbated by the general pressures of economic malfeasance and socio-economic and political duress imposed on the general population, now further exacerbated by the increasing medical tyranny being imposed under the guise of a supposed pandemic. There are plentiful examples of members of all ethnic groups who believed in and fought for human equality and gender equality, that occur throughout history and even at present, that reveal such ideas as ludicrous. Such, ideas, being false, do not help the cause of morality, ethics, understanding, and social harmony. Rather, they actually undergird feelings of resentment, hatred, fear, anxiety, mistrust, and hostility.

Such ideas, as "white people are racist simply by being born white" are racist in themselves since they support and legitimize the false notion of the existence of "human races" and thereby absolve the power elite supported and directed institutional racism. The institutional racism that is allowed by the power elite and their technocracy and bureaucracy is because of the leaders of society, the authorities appointed by the power elite, allowing people to maintain, propagate and pass on racist ideas and allow those ideas (that are unconsciously held in the populous mind and which influence feelings and actions) to be implemented overtly or subliminally[107] as

---

[107] Existing or functioning below the threshold of the conscious mind.

institutional and corporate policies that automatically have the effect of relegating certain jobs, political positions and forms of wealth along "racial" lines instead of along ethical and moral non-discriminating lines. Yet there are some who profess the deluded ideas of whites being racist simply because they are white and even would like this taught in schools. The deluded aforesaid notion of innate white racism disregards the real issue of racism as a learned social behavior, that all members of the society are taught, that supports racist institutions, which is the real problem of society.

People who consider themselves as part of a "race" of humans that is different from other humans who are "not of their race" are following a racist belief system that supports racism. Since it is scientifically demonstrated, and therefore a fact, that there are no races and that there is only one human race and since it is also true that skin color is not a real racial differentiating physiological factor but only a superficial appearance effect of geography and the level of solar exposure, then it follows that, people who consider themselves as "blacks" or "whites", or as a "different" "kind" of "human" from other "kinds" of "humans", are following racist mindsets, not realizing that in not denying the falsehood of race they are engaging in willful ignorance as well as practicing and supporting racism and the agenda of those who seek to manipulate racists. Anyone who denies the racism of their ancestors, and that their current standard of living benefitted from that racism of the past, is complicit with the racism of the past and present by not acknowledging what occurred and not seeking to redress the wrongs of the past. In this context those and their progeny, who benefitted from past racist social actions such as slavery and the later Jim Crow prevention of the progress of "non-white" peoples, but who deny their privilege due to the advantages gained by enslaving or causing others to be held back in society while they and their families advanced, are practicing and maintaining racial injustice and racial divisions (racism) as well as a pathological delusion up to the modern era.

FROM FEUDALISM TO NEO-FEUDALISM

How the Great Recession Bank Rescue Profited The Wealthy And Hurt Lower Income People[108]

The banks and the wealthy corporations, who are first able to use the currency created by the central bank (FED) (Federal Reserve Bank is the largest bank in the world representing the worldwide wealthy power elite) are able to use that currency to buy real assets like real estate, essentially for free [so the wealthy give the funds to themselves first]. That prices out the ordinary people who need to work for their currency and save it to be able to buy assets. This issue is called "CANTILLON EFFECT". People with access to "currency" first competing with people that do not have free money will overwhelm the ones without access to the funds. The ordinary person will not be able to own property and will be forced to rent. Since they cannot acquire assets and accumulate wealth they will permanently stay in a servile position, in other words, as servants to the land lords. This *Cantillon effect* along with the slow stealing of wealth through currency inflation means that the masses will always be impoverished while the wealthy will gain their wealth and remain in a position of economic power. Economic power in the corrupt fascist system of government and economics means they will also remain in positions of power, hence the creation of a neo-feudal society with a permanent unelected ruling class and a permanent underclass.

DEFFINITIONS OF FEUDALISM:
    feu•dal•ism fyood′l-ĭz″əm: Based on the possession of all land in fief or fee and the associated link of lord to vassal, and marked by homage, legal and military duty of tenants, and forfeiture, a political and economic system of Europe from the 9th until around the 15th century.
    feudalism From medieval times, this phrase was used to define the social order in Europe. The system essentially consisted of a population of unarmed peasants who were submissive to noblemen and warriors.
    Feudalism was a system in which people gave up their own freedoms in exchange for security. According to Marxist theory, feudalism leads to capitalism, which leads to socialism. The only way to put an end to feudalism was through land reform.

---

[108] https://www.forbes.com/sites/eriksherman/2019/08/30/how-great-recession-bank-rescue-profited-the-wealthy-and-hurt-lower-income-people/?sh=6e177fdd54e6

Neo-feudalism is the present day return to feudal peasant and lord relationships. In modern times the lords are corporations and the people running them. In neo-feudalism, the tyrannical surveillance police state technocracy workers are the enforcers for the lords (rich power elites) and the peasants are the masses who will not own but will rent. In this context, neo-feudalism can be equated to the dire visions of authors George Orwell and Aldus Huxley envisioned. Thus, feudalism led to capitalism and capitalism led to fascism and fascism is now leading to neo-feudalism.

> "There are two roads travelled by humankind, those who seek to live MAAT and those who seek to satisfy their animal passions."
> –Ancient Egyptian Proverb

According to the Ancient Egyptian wisdom proverb, there are two basic personalities, or ways of human behavior, ethical and animalistic. We could explain the Ancient Egyptian concept in the context of the present-day conflict of **Maat V. Fascism and the Police State**. In this context, there are those people who see the humanity in human beings and there are others who see humanity as a herd of animals to be exploited, in other words, Human rights vs feudalism. The Human rights group advocates human rights, freedom and self-determination with personal sovereignty through recognition of the common spiritual origin of humanity. The feudalism supporting group has the megalomaniacal desire to take over the world and run it their way for their benefit and power[109] through propaganda, corruption, and coercion. Covid 19 is the intended opportunity[110] being used in the war of information and perception, propaganda and censorship, manufactured fear, paranoia, and coercion. Thus, the primary battlefields of the war being waged by the power elite are banking/wall street (national malfeasance), business, and real estate (destruction of the economy and means for the population to gain wealth so that the wealth can be acquired by the power elite institutions and he masses end up destitute debt slaves), and most importantly social media and mainstream media. This group includes the sociopaths and the power elite personalities and those suffering from "rapacious greed disorder" (greed overwhelms personalities that may not be full-blown sociopaths but who are sufficiently degraded to have their empathic and ethical capacities compromised and overwhelmed). We may consider the existence of a third group, those who are neither tending towards high ethics or excessive greed but a mixture of both founded in

---

[109] https://brandnewtube.com/watch/we-are-the-resistance-and-we-will-win-this-war_yz96TU5OWcAKIEC.html
[110] **COVID-19: THE GREAT RESET**
by Klaus Schwab and Thierry Malleret

personal egoistic self-interest; they are therefore ignorant about the higher personalities manipulating society, they are ignorant about basic facts of social life, ignorant about their rights and duties in a viable society, or they are oblivious and therefore susceptible to manipulations, like the "Fear Appeal", coming from the feudalism group. The ignorant and weak-willed masses serve as slaves to the social and economic delusions imposed on them and thereby they become victims of feudalism.[111] The feudalism advocates may also have a new agenda, depopulation. Power elite personalities such as Bill Gates, and others, have intimated that there is a need for reducing the population of the planet because the population has grown too large for the planet. This reasoning, sociopathic as it is, has been put forth as the justification for the necessity, in their rationalization, of secretly including sterility drugs in vaccines.[112]

In Western Culture, the Enlightenment movement was part of a breakdown in the feudal system of society. Capitalism ultimately replaced feudalism and proved to be a more powerful tool of enslavement but, according to the feudalism proponents, too many people became wealthier and populations grew too much so it became necessary to reign in the wealth of population. This was accomplished with the creation of central banks and fractional banking systems. Now the need, according to the globalist power elite feudalism proponents, is to cull the population, as one would do to a herd of cattle. When the United States of America was formed, some ideas of the Enlightenment, as well as some ideas from the Native American Iroquois Confederation, led to inclusion in the US constitution, some notions about human rights and nation state sovereignty that were included as federalism (national government) and state rights (state government). In Europe, the idea of a European Union was apparently conceived by the United States CIA as a plan to have an overall federal system that could control many nation-states but without as much political or legal protection for human and state rights. In Europe, there is a European Commission, which is like the presidential branch (unelected executive power), and a European Parliament, which is like the US national congress. The European Commission has most if not all the power and therefore the elected parliament is impotent. Therefore, controlling the commission affords control over all the nation states in the European Union who have joined the union. In the USA the states, according to the US constitution, have more power to resist or reject the national government dictates that are not outlined in the US constitution. So the power of the US national government

---

[111] *Who Are We?: The Challenges to America's National Identity* by Samuel P. Huntington
[112] https://pubmed.ncbi.nlm.nih.gov/12346214/

usually is exercised through coercion and bribery; but ordinary people have more power to counter that if they confront, as a united state population, the corrupt national politicians which are bought by the power elites and corporate entities. Thus, the globalist power elites have run into a problem trying to control some nations including the USA since some of the states in the USA have and are refusing the agenda of neo-feudalism and are also refusing to obey the dictates of the medical mafia. Another complication, for the power elites, has been the internet (hence the need for censorship and cancel culture), wherein alternative information to the power elite propaganda, has been disseminated, leading to many people not accepting the baseless face mask, social distancing, lockdowns, and chemical gene therapies called vaccines. Another complication for the power elites was the discovery that the drug ivermectin was found to be efficacious and safe as a treatment for whatever the "corona virus/covid 19 disease" might be. These complications have, so far, thrown a wrench in the power elite's plan to easily exert absolute control and force the fear and control on the world population and even slowing down the acceptance of the chemical gene therapies referred to as "vaccines". If expanded and supported the efforts to counter the power elite plans may prove to be a basis or foundation for a united front against the forces pushing feudalism, enslavement, and anti-human rights.

THE DELUSION (INCAPACITY AND OR UNWILLINGNESS TO FACE THE TRUTH) OF TERROR VS. SECURITY AND HUMANITARIANISM.

Another delusion suffered by the population of barbarous, propagandized, and dumbed down societies, like that of western cultures and the USA, is the delusion of believing power elite leaders when they say they are promoting democracy, security, and or humanitarianism by imposing draconian regulations supposedly to promote health and security from, for example, the supposed coronavirus pandemic or when they say then need to invade some country "over there" so we don't have to "fight them over here", etc. This is the imposition of the terror of fear. That fear tactic worked after the 9/11/01 attack on USA sites supposedly from external enemies of the USA who supposedly did not attack because they were resisting USA invasions and attacks on their country from the USA, but rather because they hated the "American way of life" supposedly implying freedom and democracy, neither of which are enjoyed by the USA population, which now lives in a surveillance state (there is no freedom without privacy); and as the Princeton study showed in the report entitled: "U.S. No Longer An Actual Democracy".[113]

In this context terrorism is the imposition of control and inhumane, exploitative regulations or life inhibiting policies on a population. ***In the year 2020,*** a new version of social terrorism was imposed with the regulations supposedly to prevent the spread of covid 19 coronavirus disease. Even though after months of peer-reviewed studies being conducted throughout the year, showing that mask-wearing, social distancing, and lockdowns have no discernible positive effect when imposed on the general asymptomatic members of the population but rather had deleterious effects on health, the power elite continued and still continue to impose such regulations and even tried to double down on those regulations by forcing people to wear not just one ineffective mask that actually has physiological negative effects that suppress the immune system, but started talking about forcing people to wear two masks, along with continued social distancing and lockdowns, even after taking a vaccine, etc.[114] Later it was revealed that the policy of "vaccinated" people in the media and in government and by the supposed health officials like Fauci were continuing to wear masks in public and when on television so as to maintain the façade of the pandemic scare.

FAUCI ADMITS WEARING A MASK WHILE FULLY VACCINATED WAS POLITICAL THEATER[115]

This is the continued imposition of the "Fear Appeal" terror tactic along with giving people actions to do (like mask wearing-again, which has been proven to be ineffective) so they may feel they are complying and doing something to help themselves. In reality, they are harming their own health of body[116], and also of mind while submitting their sovereignty and wealth

---

[113] PRINCETON STUDY: U.S. NO LONGER AN ACTUAL DEMOCRACY- APRIL 18, 2014
https://talkingpointsmemo.com/livewire/princeton-experts-say-us-no-longer-democracy
[114] https://www.cdc.gov/media/releases/2021/p0130-requires-face-masks.html
Update-In early 2021 the CDC issued guidelines to recommend people who are vaccinated to stop wearing masks indoors – so as to entice others to get vaccinated and get back their freedoms
[115] https://thefederalist.com/2021/05/18/fauci-admits-wearing-a-mask-while-fully-vaccinated-was-political-theater/
[116] https://medium.com/theusareviewer/the-potential-dangers-of-wearing-a-face-mask-51b9b86980a
https://www.jennifermargulis.net/wearing-mask-can-harm-your-health/

to supposed authorities. Additionally, at the same time, they are living the lie of not facing the truth of the falsehood of the mandates and taking appropriate actions to promote real health and ethical actions to resist the imposition of inhumane regulations. Those inhumane regulations lead to physical and mental diseases. On 1/20/21 Dr. Muata Ashby conducted a study comparing the deaths per 100 thousand people in each of the states of the USA. The result was that the states without mask-wearing mandates had fewer deaths attributed to coronavirus than the states that had mask-wearing mandates.[117] This finding confirms that the mask-wearing mandates are wrong and should be stopped immediately. This confirms the earlier findings by other researchers.

1 in 6 Americans Went Into Therapy for the First Time in 2020
Analysis by Dr. Joseph Mercola[118]
Story at-a-glance

THE DELUSION (INCAPACITY AND OR UNWILLINGNESS TO FACE THE TRUTH OF) OF DEMOCRACY VS. FASCISM.

The delusion (incapacity and or unwillingness, of the society, to face the truth of) of democracy vs. fascism is the incapacity to realize that one does not live in a democracy, despite the constant claim by news reporters and politicians that the USA has and is founded on a democratic system of politics. The USA was founded with a constitutional republic system. The founding fathers were afraid of direct democracy and thus created a system of representative politics so that the power elite of the society would be able to maintain control of the political system while deluding the population into believing that they have power over their political and economic lives. The public only has the power to elect which power elite appointed politicians they want but have no power to change the system of government or economy. Of course, if there was any doubt about

---

https://althealthworks.com/doctors-warn-potential-long-term-side-effects-of-mask-wearing-include-shortness-of-breath-a-weakened-immune-system-and-chronic-respiratory-conditions/
[117] https://usafacts.org/visualizations/coronavirus-covid-19-spread-map/
https://www.mercurynews.com/2020/11/10/these-are-the-15-states-that-dont-require-masks/
[118] https://articles.mercola.com/sites/articles/archive/2021/02/04/covid-19-pandemic-mental-health.aspx?ui=152220df1deda081f73727bc10a8407027b248ba493a7ce71f4a1e73a6c1d882&cid_source=dnl&cid_medium=email&cid_content=art2HL&cid=20210204&mid=DM794933&rid=1075905019

the nature of the political system the Princeton Study[119] as well as the most well-known politicians, former president Jimmy Carter,[120] have demonstrated and asserted that the USA does not have democracy (majority rule) and in fact also does not have a representative system because there is no representation that responds to the needs and desires of the general population; it responds only to the corporatocracy and the power elite that have bribed the politicians and have bought them off. This is a description of fascism. Thus, the system called "democracy" may be considered as a euphemism and more accurately as a façade of fascism.

> Former President Jimmy Carter was again critical of the National Security Agency surveillance program brought to light by fugitive leaker Edward Snowden. [121]
> "America has no functioning democracy at this moment," Carter said at a closed-door event in Atlanta covered by a German newsmagazine.

THE DELUSION ABOUT CAPITALISM VERSUS EQUAL OPPORTUNITY.

The delusion (mental deficiency due, in part, to incapacity and or unwillingness to face the truth) of capitalism vs. equal opportunity in society is the belief system that the western-style governments, especially that of the USA, are superior to any others and this idea is conflated with the economic system of capitalism, as a supposed system that can enrich the society, which is treated almost as sacrosanct, at least in the media propaganda, and the constant statements by politicians and corporate leaders, who, of course, have the most to gain from keeping and maintaining a system of "democracy", which is demonstrably not democratic but instead fascistic, and also maintain the system of capitalism that has blossomed into fascism and oligarchy controlled by a plutocrat group of global power elite individuals. The belief (delusion), of the lower classes (everyone other than the power elite), in the façade of democracy and capitalism, that are in

---

[119] **PRINCETON STUDY: U.S. NO LONGER AN ACTUAL DEMOCRACY- APRIL 18, 2014**
https://talkingpointsmemo.com/livewire/princeton-experts-say-us-no-longer-democracy
[120] **JIMMY CARTER IS CORRECT THAT THE U.S. IS NO LONGER A DEMOCRACY 08/03/2015 11:48 AM ET UPDATED AUG 03, 2016**
HTTPS://WWW.HUFFPOST.COM/ENTRY/JIMMY-CARTER-IS-CORRECT-T_B_7922788
[121] https://www.upi.com/blog/2013/07/18/Jimmy-Carter-on-NSA-America-has-no-functioning-democracy/6541374165224/

reality totalitarianism and barbarism, allows those systems to be upheld by that power elite as virtues and allows the general masses to believe in them even as they are demonstrably false as evidenced by the extreme inequality that has been produced by their adoption. The belief, by the lower classes, continues despite how the political system openly serves the desires of the power elite and if at all provides anything to the masses those are only subsistence level services. The rest of the population are seen as fodder for commodification, that is, treated and manipulated into becoming objects for the commercial benefit of corporations; otherwise they are seen and or treated as liabilities to the corporate state, that needs to employ greater and greater means of surveillance and violence to control them, given the unrest caused by disparities that have been produced due to the same economic inequalities brought on by the rapacious, power-hungry power elite policies that were enacted by the politicians and enforced by their technocrats and bureaucrats (police, courts, government agencies, etc.), that manage the society for them.

POLITICAL INTOLERANCE, "WOKE CULTURE", "MEETOO", "MILLENNIAL FRAGILITY" AND "CANCEL CULTURE" BLOSSOMING INTO FULL BLOWN CORPORATE AND GOVERNMENT ENDORSED CENSORSHIP.

In the 21st century many past social maladies that had existed, in previous decades, at more manageable levels, have arisen in a manner that has deteriorated society and enhanced the power elite's capacity to manipulate and exploit the masses. "Woke culture", in its highest context, might have been thought of as a description of being aware and awake to the situation of life in order to face it and make the best decisions possible. The "MeToo" movement might have been thought of as standing up and facing down the chauvinist and paternalistic, abusiveness in general society specifically, though not exclusively directed against women. "Millennial Fragility" may be thought of as a condition exhibited in the younger generation, though not exclusively, by young people, of being incapable of handling criticism, inconvenience, hard work, and overall stress.

The political intolerance that seems to have begun, in earnest, during the Ronald Reagan era, with republican party politicians taking advantage of prior year progressive gains against racism, seized on the fears of mostly southerners and non-urban dwellers and stoked those fears in order to gain adherents into coalitions comprised of those fearful of cultural changes, latent and or overt racist tendencies, social conservatives, religious fundamentalists and corporate sponsors. These politicians developed into an acerbic philosophical conservative movement of taking no prisoners, no compromise, and no negotiation or friendship with those who disagree with them. Thus, was fomented polarization, hatred, and vitriol in politics that reflected back onto the base, the followers of the party in cities and towns across the country and was reinforced by the echo chamber of repeated vitriolic and extreme statements in talk radio and later cable "news" channels, like Fox News and MSNBC, that led to the present situation of incapacity of ordinary people, even in the same family, to communicate on areas of political disagreement.

"Astro-turf (front groups run by lobbyists and corporate interests) groups like the moral majority and the tea-party were created so that people with such feelings (fear, racism, conservative religious, anger, etc.) could coalesce around them and be politically manipulated. The republican party vitriol tactic of virtue signaling, identity politics, and corrupt negotiation in bad faith came to its height in the 1990s with the takeover of congress by the republican party under the direction of Newton Gingrich and has remained as rapacious, vitriolic, argumentative, and unethical ever since, also corrupting what was left of any semblance of ethics and traditional liberalism in the democratic party (which was already compromised by the corruption due to its own corporate takeover that was ushered in by president Bill Clinton and democrat party leaders in congress). This state of social consciousness facilitates authoritarianism in a winner take all political structure; this leads to a totalitarian approach by the political parties that is blindly supported by the party's followers (including party operatives and ordinary citizens that remain deluded about party politics as a means either to promote real democracy or egoistically getting their political desires fulfilled. The power elite does not care about democracy or fulfilling the desires of citizens; it only cares about using them to gain more wealth, exert more control and stay in power with the façade of a democratic process. With each new election, the winning party becomes more authoritarian, commits more immoral and illegal acts, domestically and internationally, with impunity, as more people become increasingly frustrated and apathetic about politics, even as some become more hardened in their political support of their party and condone whatever may be done to the opposition, their fellow citizens with a different belief.

Amidst the political mayhem, the social movements within the population, seeking redress for past wrongs, the *woke culture*, *MeeToo*, and the breakdown of culture leading to psychological fragility and overall frustration open the door for exploring varied means of satisfaction, but not in a mature and educated manner, but rather in the manner of unhinged emotional flailing without direction in combination with egoistic desire and feelings of victimization that have given way to *cancel culture* which is blossoming into full-blown and government identity politics and government endorsed censorship, which is encouraged or forced on media corporations by corruption, coercion or duress. In this way, woke culture, MeeToo, and the breakdown of culture leading to psychological fragility, which are dysfunctional reactions and dysfunctional adaptations to injustices or social maladies (disease), become foci for individuals to direct their emotional reactions based on the pains suffered but the direction is towards illusory perceived sources of causes of the suffering and not the true source of the pain. The true source of the pain is the corrupt leadership that has allowed and which benefits from the injustices to exist and persist in society. For example, protesting to get justice by having one police officer jailed for killing a person does not fix the issue of institutional racism and institutional police militarization and criminal impunity. So, if street protests do not transform into real political and legal change the legal system and the political class continue unabated and the suffering will continue and increase.

Cancel culture developed in recent years as a socially acceptable form of censorship and forceful movement to stop any opposing view that was found to be hurtful or insulting by the person(s) seeking its cancellation. So extreme is the idea as to cancel anyone even preemptively, for saying anything the listener does not want to hear, regardless of it if is true or not. In this context cancel culture is a dysfunctional coping mechanism or an immature coping mechanism for people who cannot handle hearing anything their deluded, immature offended, or fragile personality cannot take. This situation of the development and increasing occurrence of fragile personalities in the society, is of course, due to faulty parenting in the form of biological parents who grew up as degraded personalities themselves, working and trying to survive in the rat race world created by the power elite, and because of the ignorant, rapacious and vitriolic social leadership in the form of sociopathic criminal presidents, and congresspeople. Instead of canceling others, which represses thoughts, feelings, and desires and promotes mental complexes and social aberrant behaviors, they should be allowed all speech, and this will allow the irrational, stupid, foolish, or corrupt speech to reveal itself in the court of public consideration and open discussion so as to receive due consideration and resolution in the form of dismissal if found to be unsound, therapy if needed, or further consideration and proper response in the form of accommodation and or wider social change, thereby showing the speaker caring and due consideration of their concerns, which promotes resolution and healing for the individual and harmony, as well as positive progress, for the society. The cancel culture causes repression and supports the fragility of the personality, both of which lead to greater and intensifying personality disorders and pathologies. Private groups and government agencies have adopted the cancel culture tactic as a means to justify leaning on media corporations to follow suit, thereby increasing identity politics, heightened emotions and virtue signaling thereby damaging or incapacitating thoughtful discussion and free speech against them as a means to impose the desired agendas without intellectual opposition and with blind emotional assistance by ignorant or deluded followers.

People like George Carlin would not be allowed to speak on many college campuses, in our present times, as the students themselves, having ignorantly adopted the misguided application of the ideas of "Woke culture, "MeToo", "Millennial Fragility" and social justice advocates, coupled with miseducation (wrong parenting and or socialization and or conditioning by the corrupt mainstream media, corrupt social media, and corrupt political pundits) and psychological fragility, prevent anyone who will speak to them about their own failings and the mature and more effective means to achieve their goals – if people do not speak in a way and in agreement with their notions of reality based on their opinions and feelings; this as if their opinions and feelings matter more than facts or objective reality or the feelings and opinions of others. Such is the state of the dysfunctional culture that is not able to reflect thoughtfully on issues because the minds are egoistic, ignorant, deluded, and their intellects are atrophied and they operate mostly at a crippled emotional level that cannot be considered as an adult in the context of previous generations' capacity to face individual and collective challenges of life. Such a sizable degraded segment of population in a society can be easily manipulated by demagogues and media propagandists (news anchors, and pundits) as it is not a large step to move from demanding the cancellation of some individuals to being satisfied when one's political party, in control of the government, actively advocate for or passively allow people to be deplatformed by independent groups, or corporations, essentially canceling their speech from the social arena; indeed this is what is happening, censorship, not overtly from government institutions but by encouraging or coercing social groups, businesses, and social media companies to do the censorship.

The prevailing government in the USA (democratic party), holding the reins on social media companies or rather in collusion with them, allows them to deplatform and or ban certain people's words and works under the guise of protecting society from them. Even though the cancel culture, blossoming into full-blown censorship, occurs in a society frustrated by decades of political fascism and oligarchy as well as economic disparity and financial sector, political, and corporate frauds, mainstream medial lies and propaganda, banking frauds, constant wars, medical frauds, etc. that have impoverished the population. Still the population acts out, not to confront those issues but flails in the direction of seeking supposed social justice against lesser and sometimes inconsequential issues, the symptoms of social, political and economic problems of the society. Thus, such a population is incapable of confronting the source of even their own disempowerment, impoverishment, abuse, and mistreatment. The main source of the problem of such a population is the holding on to the lies that individuals and society as a whole tell themselves. Those lies emasculate the individuals from being able to see the manipulations, the dumbing down of the population, and the perpetration of intentional frauds, not mistakes, by the political and corporate classes, which only seek their own wellbeing and power. Seeking redress in the society by protesting against the social symptoms of the problem of the power elite, which manifests as fascism, corporatocracy and the fascist surveillance police state, etc. is like seeking the solution to a local flood while not fixing the broken dam upstream and always remaining in a state of emergency, bailing out the water and never being thoughtful, looking for the source of the problem causing the continuous floods. Real and effective action would mean going upstream to the person in charge and impeaching them for their willful negligence and intentional harm that they perpetrated on society and instituting a system whereby such personalities cannot get into positions of power and cause society-wide harm; otherwise, it is the Stockholm syndrome being played out on the grand scale of an entire society that is captive and held hostage by the sociopathic overlords (government authorities, corporate heads, media opinion leaders and their handlers, the power elite) and their

Orwellian newspeak[122], memes, and slogans professing freedom and justice but yet delivering oppression, corruption, fear, disease, and suffering. Those sociopathic overlords have appointed themselves as authorities through corrupt electoral and media systems, spouting the words of democracy, progress, togetherness, and social unity while implementing intentional error and irrational policies that always seem to accidentally lead to wars, make them richer, impoverish the society at large and cause mayhem and division in the culture.

CURRENT DAY COMMON EXAMPLES OF POWER ELITE FASCISM IN THE USA AND ABROAD:

The year 2020 revealed naked, open, unapologetic statements and ruthless acts of fascism and terrorism against the USA population and populations abroad That fascism and terrorism was implemented with the imposition of an unknown virus fabricated pandemic, lockdowns, propaganda, and censorship along with coup d'états and destabilizations of foreign governments.

FASCISM may be defined as a government controlled by Power Elites, plutocrats[123] oligarchs[124] through their corporate entities and enterprises, corporate media, and owned government officials working together. They use the instrumentalities and powers of the legislative, judicial, and executive powers of the government apparatus to override national and international elections, laws, and apply those to undermine personal and national sovereignties towards the goal of acquiring power and impoverishing populations. This is the corporatist power elite ideology of world order and domination. This is the ideology that has and is in control of western supposed democratic countries and eastern supposed communist countries as well as dictatorships around the world. So, the same power elite ideology of world control and domination can and does at present, operate

---

[122] Prof. Jerry Kroth ropaganda and Manipulation: How mass media engineers and distorts our perceptions   https://youtu.be/Pfo5gPG72KM

[123] A plutocracy or plutarchy is a society that is ruled or controlled by people of great wealth or income.

[124] **Oligarchy** (from Greek ὀλιγαρχία (oligarkhía); from ὀλίγος (olígos) 'few', and ἄρχω (arkho) 'to rule or to command') is a form of power structure in which power rests with a small number of people.

in the democratic, communist, right-wing, left-wing, or autocratic governments alike.

Example #1: Mainstream Media and Social Media Tech companies practicing censorship on behalf of the ruling elite (the neoliberal establishment in control of the democratic party, those who control government and banking) and the government policies that support their paradigm for society.

> *The New Domestic War on Terror is Coming.* "No speculation is needed. Those who wield power are demanding it. The only question is how much opposition they will encounter."
> -by Glen Greenwald January 21, 2021

Donald Trump lost the presidential election in the Fall of 2020. Many people who feel appalled by the personality of Donald Trump and his followers and by extension those who voted for him, and also the right-wing groups in general, feel it is right that he and his followers be censored for what is considered vulgar violent supporting hate speech, rhetoric supporting racism, sexism, etc. When there were democratic party presidents in office the republicans and their followers expressed similar desires and feelings against the democrats. However, what may not be reflected upon in the heat of disgust and the preening stance of electoral victory (by the neoliberal establishment in control of the democratic party (those who now control government) and banking) is the factor that just as the subversive tactics of the USA government and armed forces were and still are used against other countries and then were later used, though groups such as the CIA[125] to subvert the USA media, using them to silence opponents, for the benefit of the ruling party, the prison industrial complex, the federal reserve banking cartel, the pharmaceutical industrial complex, and the big tech industrial complex; now we see those same corruptions being used against the USA population.

"We'll know our disinformation program is complete when everything the American public believes is false."
- William Casey, CIA Director at first staff meeting 1981

Censorship may be used against the right-leaning population and those who are Trump supporters now but will eventually be used against anyone even

---

[125] See the Church Report – congressional investigation uncovering evidence of the Central Intelligence Agency subversion of the USA mainstream media

on the left, who does not conform to the power structure narratives of the prevailing neoliberal ideology[126] dominating the USA democratic party. The power structure narratives are not partisan but rather use parties to achieve their goals, so they are supra-partisan and indeed supra-national. When people are acting out of emotional or personal fear, angst, or revenge, etc., that serves to perpetuate injustices that, though they may be visited on others and that makes one feel emotionally satisfied, in the short term, it acts to corrode the ethical conscience and fabric of a sane and balanced society in the long run. This means that the same acts that were perpetrated on others are visited upon oneself.

This occurrence, of one's actions having a cause and effect result that reflects back on oneself or on the same society, is a classical Maatian wisdom tenet. In this equation, of external acts coming back and affecting the actor, from the standpoint of MAAT PHILOSOPHY, it also means that one is responsible for the social ills that were supported and or visited upon others, for one's material or emotional short-term satisfaction as well as the consequences of long-term damage and suffering, for oneself and others, that will ensue.

The following is an example, from January 2021, of censorship being used by (the neoliberal establishment in control of the democratic party (those who control government) and turned on left-wing groups. This shows that the censorship is not just being directed, from the democratic party leaders and followers, towards right-wing republican party groups such as the followers of Donald Trump, or that it is being directed for ethical reasons or for the protection of society or to promote more civil discourse. The purpose is to squelch all dissenting points of view, especially those that might gain traction and coalesce significant opposition in the population, regardless of if they come from republicans or democrats or from any other political party or non-political group, that contradict the messages and authority of the fascist government controlled by the corporate global power elite.

> According to economist Joseph Stiglitz, there has been a severe increase in market power of corporations, largely due to U.S. antitrust laws being weakened by neoliberal reforms, leading to growing income inequality and a generally underperforming economy.[127] He states that to improve

---

[126] neoliberal ideology may be understood as a political manifestation of totalitarian fascism
[127] *Stiglitz, Joseph (May 13, 2019). "Three decades of neoliberal policies have decimated the middle class, our economy, and our democracy". MarketWatch. Retrieved August 22, 2019.*

the economy, it is necessary to decrease the influence of money on U.S. politics.[128]

In 2013, economist Edmund Phelps criticized the economic system of the U.S. and other western countries in recent decades as being what he calls "the new corporatism", which he characterizes as a system in which the state is far too involved in the economy, tasked with "protecting everyone against everyone else", but in which at the same time big companies have a great deal of influence on the government, with lobbyists' suggestions being "welcome, especially if they come with bribes".[129]

Economist Jeffrey Sachs described the United States as a corporatocracy in *The Price of Civilization* (2011).[10] He suggested that it arose from four trends: weak national parties and strong political representation of individual districts, the large U.S. military establishment after World War II, large corporations using money to finance election campaigns, and globalization tilting the balance of power away from workers.[130]

Twitter Admits To Censoring Criticism of The Indian Government[131]

April 25, 2021

==========================

Facebook deletes 120,000-member group where people posted stories of alleged adverse vaccine reactions[132]

April 26, 2021

==========================

Facebook Bans Left Party Without Explanation.[133]

---

[128] *Stiglitz, Joseph (October 23, 2017). "America Has a Monopoly Problem—and It's Huge". The Nation. Retrieved August 22, 2019.*

[129] Phelps, Edmund (2013). *Mass Flourishing. How grassroots innovation created jobs, challenge, and change (1st edition).* Princeton: Princeton University Press. Chapter 6, section 4: *The New Corporatism.*

[130] *Sachs, Jeffrey (2011). The Price of Civilization. New York: Random House. pp. 105, 106, 107. ISBN 978-1-4000-6841-8.*

[131] https://jonathanturley.org/2021/04/25/twitter-admits-to-censoring-criticism-of-the-indian-government/

[132] https://www.naturalnews.com/2021-04-26-facebook-deletes-120000-member-group-vaccine-adverse-reactions.html

[133] https://youtu.be/DKHFWBd5EIw

Those who could be considered as "populist" leaders would antagonize the fascist establishment and therefore would receive most harassment, deplatforming, censorship, imprisonment, and threats to their life. In the example above, already in January 2021, the censorship was turning not just towards right-wing or republican groups, but on left-wing groups, showing that the prevailing democratic party is not ideologically aligned with traditional liberal or democratic norms, but rather with a fascist, totalitarian, neoliberal agenda. This state of affairs, the party in power tacitly approving censorship by supposedly private corporations (Facebook, Twitter, Youtube, etc.), may be seen as the corporate component of fascist government; so it may be referred to as corporatocracy[134]; indeed, fascism may be thought of as corporatism, the collusion of government officials with their corporate controllers for the purpose of curtailing the liberty and wealth of the individual and promoting profits and power for corporations. This is accomplished by uniting and coordinating government state power and corporate power against individual freedom and individual and national sovereignty for control and exploitation of individuals and nations.

Characteristics of Corporatocracy (Corporatism) and Fascism:

> Historian Howard Zinn argues that during the Gilded Age in the United States, the U.S. government was acting exactly as Karl Marx described capitalist states: "pretending neutrality to maintain order, but serving the interests of the rich".[135]

========

> "Fascism should more appropriately be called Corporatism because it is a merger of state and corporate power"
> ..."The definition of fascism is The marriage of corporation and state"
> ...The Fascist State organizes the nation, but leaves a sufficient margin of liberty to the individual; the latter is deprived of all useless and possibly harmful freedom, but retains what is essential; the deciding power in this question cannot be the individual, but the State alone....
> — Benito Mussolini

---

[134] Rule by an oligarchy of corporate elites through the manipulation of a formal democracy.
[135] *Zinn, Howard (2005). A People's History of the United States. New York: Harper Perennial Modern Classics. p. 258. ISBN 978-0-06-083865-2.*

Example #2 Elon Musk

'We will coup whoever we want': Elon Musk sparks online riot with quip about overthrow of Bolivia's Evo Morales

Elon Musk openly expressed support for the subversion of the government of Bolivia for the benefit (take resources from another country) of himself and his company. Fascism was on full display as the US government officials and covert agents collude with local opposition officials to overthrow the current president who was protecting the country's resources for its people.[136]

Example #3 Jeff Bezos, AMAZON and the CIA[137]

Amazon to take Parler offline
-January 9, 2021

Parler CEO says app will be offline 'longer than expected' because of Amazon, Apple and Google[138]

The AMAZON digital service, and other tech companies, AWS, that hosted the social media company, PARLER (www.parler.com), on their servers, suddenly dropped PARLER, in a coordinated fashion; all refused to host PARLER. At the behest of many politicians in congress advocating censorship of supposed anti-American (really means anti-

---

[136] https://www.rt.com/news/495820-musk-coup-bolivia-lithium-tesla/
https://www.youtube.com/results?search_query=we+will+coup+whoever+we+want+elon+musk
https://youtu.be/vc2SA0--uiA

[137] https://www.huffpost.com/entry/the-cia-amazon-bezos-and_b_4559317
http://www.camelotdaily.com/cia-funded-amazon-ceo-jeff-bezos-parties-with-fmr-jewish-goldman-sachs-ceo-lloyd-blankfein-google-funded-josh-kushner-brother-of-jared-kushner-aboard-jewish-homosexual-billionaire-david-geffens-s/
https://www.worldtribune.com/bezos-internet-cloud-deal-with-the-cia-worth-twice-what-he-paid-for-the-washington-post/

[138] Published Mon, Jan 11 2021 5:14 AM EST Updated Tue, Jan 12 2021 6:06 AM EST
https://www.cnbc.com/2021/01/11/parler-drops-offline-after-amazon-withdraws-support.html

government) speech and sentiments, Jeff Bezos, the owner of AMAZON, which has contracts with the CIA (government), the surveillance industrial complex and who also purchased a prominent newspaper de-platformed PARLER, a free self-styled speech web site, so it could not function on AMAZON servers.[139] Amazon cited the reason for the deplatforming on supposed posts that incite violence; however, Facebook has also been accused of similar posts but has not been taken down.[140] Then, other corporations followed AMAZON's actions and denied PARLER the opportunity to get hosted with them so that PARLER could go online. So, for Facebook, there is acceptance, since they support the government narratives, and for PARLER there was no opportunity for disputing or fixing any complaints but rather there is the immediate obliteration of PARLER, which was the only alternative to facebook –because it hosts alternative views to those held by the neoliberal corporate power elite establishment. Without free speech in a supposedly free society, especially in an environment of exploitation and impunity for the power elites, there will necessarily grow seething discontent that will further draw more totalitarian responses (including overt violence through police violence) from the power elites and further degradation of the society. PARLER was in direct competition with Facebook and Google, which own, manage and support Youtube, all of which practice propaganda, subliminal behavior modification, allow violent content and propaganda and censorship.[141] The power elites in control of AMAZON directed that company to remove PARLER ostensibly because of "hate speech or the incitement of violence" but PARLER, which had a reputation of promoting free speech, was in competition with the more powerful companies (facebook, twitter, etc.) that are in line with the neoliberal power elites, propaganda and censorship tactics. It is important to note that though Trump's followers started using PARLER it was not only them; many people disgusted with companies such as facebook, its censorship and psychological manipulations, CIA and NSA connections etc. moved to use that platform as a safer and more effective social media platform. The real competition was between the censoring platforms in favor of the democrat party and neoliberalism vs. PARLER which touted more free speech and attracted many non-Trump followers

---

[139] https://www.washingtontimes.com/news/2021/jan/9/amazon-take-parler-offline/
[140] **THREATS MADE OVER FACEBOOK ARE NOT ILLEGAL UNLESS INTENTIONALLY MALEVOLENT, COURT RULES**
HTTPS://WWW.INDEPENDENT.CO.UK/NEWS/WORLD/AMERICAS/THREATS-MADE-OVER-FACEBOOK-ARE-NOT-ILLEGAL-UNLESS-INTENTIONALLY-MALEVOLENT-COURT-RULES-10289724.HTML
[141] https://www.forbes.com/sites/abrambrown/2020/06/27/parlers-founder-explains-why-he-built-trumps-new-favorite-social-media-app/?sh=24c8dff95016

interested in free and non- surveilled social media as well as Trump and his populist but republican party leaning followers, after Trump saw his messages being interfered with on the more powerful platforms. His followers were for Trump and, at least in principle, if not in substance and politically effectively, in opposition to the democrats and neoliberals. In other words, many, if not most of the Trump followers were not necessarily politically savvy but supported him, even though he proved to be a fraud as he failed to pursue his campaign promises to them and instead worked for tax breaks for the elites and support of the military-industrial complex, because of visceral fears and perceived ethnic existential threats. Having no other outlet or political prospect after decades of disappointments with the political system and from both parties, many Trump supporters supported him out of those nativist fears but some out of disgust for the power structure and corrupt political system. Thus, they followed a member of the moneyed class (Trump) who spoke in the language of populist politics but in reality, was never intending or able (due to 1-he never intended to help anyone other than himself and the moneyed class, 2-opposition from the other oligarchs controlling both the democrat and republican parties) to deliver on promises to them but symbolically connected with them on that visceral level and cultivated their genuine disgust for the state of politics and some having racist and or nativist fears, in order to martial their support for electoral victory.

Other examples of corporate censorship on behalf of the current neo-liberal political interests include facebook censoring socialist left groups on behalf of themselves and the neoliberal democratic party.
objected to the narrative of the authority figures, those who viscerally mistrust and or hate authorities, especially government authorities following the democrats with their neo-liberal agenda, but who do not have evidence on the supposed virus so the objection is also based on scientific ignorance. Some of these personalities believe in gun ownership and some, but not all, may be considered as bigots and racists. The other group objects, to being forced to follow dictates from a ruling class, out of civil libertarian principles (personal sovereignty and the right to control what goes into one's body). They may also believe in evidence-based knowledge, facts about the disease that do indicate no necessity for face-masking and or lockdowns along with the discovery of effective medicines to treat the disease which also invalidates the necessity of masking, social distancing, or lockdowns. As of the beginning of the year 2021, neither group made progress in opposing the agenda of the authority figures but those in states with republican party control and or governors fared better in terms of

escaping the most draconian and "seemingly irrational" impositions by the authority figures. States such as South Dakota, Texas and Florida and countries such as Sweden, Taiwan and Japan are examples of states and countries that did not impose draconian mask mandates, social distancing, or lockdowns. The state of South Dakota never imposed any mask mandate, social distancing, or lockdowns and they fared better than many the states that did imposed and continue imposing mask mandates, social distancing, or lockdowns.

Twitter Censors Peer-Reviewed Mask Study[142]

-Analysis by Dr. Joseph Mercola

The term "irrational"[143], used earlier, is used in a context referring to those on the receiving end of the impositions, from the supposed authorities, of the mask mandates, social distancing, and lockdown policies that from the receiving end, do not make sense concerning the supposed purpose of stemming disease, because in actuality they have been found to cause more disease instead of preventing disease. However, the impositions are rational if it is considered that there is an aberrant agenda, an ulterior motive behind them, of training people to obey on command, imposing control on the population, and destroying the economy so that moneyed interests can take over the properties (like houses) and business assets in the wake of high unemployment and or bankruptcies, and people left impotent and destitute, incapable of opposing the moneyed corporate forces and their bought-off politicians. From that perspective the supposed irrational policies make sense. The draconian policies could also facilitate a suspected agenda to reset the currency system to replace the US Dollar that has lost over 97% of its value since the creation of the federal reserve bank in 1913.

The year 2020 revealed to what extent the supposed health agencies, together with drug companies and in collusion with government authority figures and the media supporting them, were willing to go to produce

---

[142] https://articles.mercola.com/sites/articles/archive/2021/04/28/twitter-censors-peer-reviewed-mask-study.aspx?ui=152220df1deda081f73727bc10a8407027b248ba493a7ce71f4a1e73a6c1d882&sd=20200829&cid_source=dnl&cid_medium=email&cid_content=art2HL&cid=20210428_HL2&mid=DM869849&rid=1144183508

[143] https://youtu.be/lL6U31QKOQc

experimental and dangerous chemical concoctions and call them "vaccines". This was done so they could avoid having those experimental therapies classified as experimental chemical therapies and thereby avoid liability for any damage or deaths that might occur as a result of their use. Considering that we have safe and effective supplements and drugs to use for coronavirus disease that have not killed or maimed anyone, those imposing the experimental gene therapies referred to as "vaccines" do not care about how many people might be killed or maimed. While most drugs that kill even less than a dozen people would have been withdrawn, as of the 5/24/2021 release of VAERS data:

Found 4,201 cases where Vaccine targets COVID-19 (COVID19) and Patient Died[144]

The year 2020 revealed how, even after the vaccines have proven to be not safe and not effective and have killed over 4000 people in the USA and more than that in Europe, most people, a majority of the population, despite the mistrust of government, political parties, and the media, were willing to obey the authority figures and submit their bodies to the experimental treatments, in essence, to be experimented on as guinea pigs. This last factor is ominous because it supports the other failed idea that the supposed health leaders are foisting, that most of the population needs to be vaccinated to attain supposed unproven vaccine-induced "herd immunity" even as some scientists are showing that herd immunity is being reached[145] without vaccines (the vaccines will get the credit for any positive results, not natural immunity); this as calls continue to go out in support of enforcing vaccinations or denying travel or the capacity to work when the lockdowns end. Other calls are going out to create travel vaccine passports and preparing rosters of those who do not vaccinate, etc. clearly leading to efforts of coercion if not outright forced vaccination including vaccinating children without their parent's consent so as to bypass the safety concerns and choice rights of parents. Vaccine Passports, even if they were constitutional, which they are not, would not protect anyone from contracting or spreading disease since the so-called chemical gene therapies that have been developed have not been proven to protect anyone from anything and in fact the only claim has been made that they *reduce*

---

[144] https://www.medalerts.org/vaersdb/findfield.php?EVENTS=on&PAGENO=1&PERPAGE=10&ESORT&REVERSESORT&VAX=%28COVID19%29&VAXTYPES=%28COVID-19%29&DIED=Yes&fbclid=IwAR2rBWzmzUUh-5eWc3N4gp6PV3aEnpIyzAX0Oazu32g8hzrPHqKfVmflV1M
[145] https://youtu.be/lL6U31QKOQc

symptoms of the infection.[146] As will be seen later on, that claim is fatally misleading.

Again, if vaccines are safe and effective for those who choose to be vaccinated why are people who do not want to be vaccinated being forced to vaccinate? Why are the legitimate safety concerns about vaccines not being answered by authorities and instead they are instead responding by trying to secretly vaccinate people?

D.C. Council approves bill allowing children to get vaccines without parents' consent
Oct. 20, 2020 at 4:11 p.m. EDT

In a positive trend, some states are moving to preclude any requirement for a "vaccine passport".[147] If this trend is successful, the total control over people's liberty and movements that is sought by the fascist power elites would fail.

Group supports NC bill prohibiting mandatory vaccine; bans businesses from requiring vaccine info[148]

---

[146] https://articles.mercola.com/sites/articles/archive/2021/05/10/the-rise-of-utilitarian-extremism.aspx?ui=152220df1deda081f73727bc10a8407027b248ba493a7ce71f4a1e73a6c1d882&sd=20200829&cid_source=dnl&cid_medium=email&cid_content=art1HL&cid=20210510&mid=DM880981&rid=1154255890

[147] https://www.ncleg.gov/BillLookUp/2021/HB%20558

[148] https://www.cbs17.com/news/north-carolina-news/group-supports-nc-bill-prohibiting-mandatory-vaccine-bans-businesses-from-requiring-vaccine-info/

CAPITALISM, FASCISM AND THE ILLUSION OF DEMOCRACY

Many people, who may consider themselves as part of the successful or aspiringly successful part of the corporate sector seemingly earnestly go on speaking tours and are readily accepted on cable news and cable business channels to profess the virtues of capitalism. When they are confronted with the contradictions, cronyism, corruption, criminality, and revolving door between corporate elites and the government agency positions, they lament that the system is broken so they say "all we need to do is reform it." Yet the reform never occurs and the law-breaking among the corporate leaders and government leaders now holds no penalty. Such a logical but flawed argument, about reforming capitalism, is usually stated by corporate heads and political leaders and their operatives, all of whom benefit from the present capitalist fascist economic and governance structure. A prime example of the crony and fascist relationship between government officials and corporations is insider trading, which is legal for congress members but illegal for ordinary citizens.

Those people in the general population, who aspire to become "rich" or to have a business or a job in a prosperous company are eager to believe such rhetoric even as decades of the implementation of capitalism has demonstrated its fatally corrosive effects on government and social institutions. In fact, those people are being duped by the corporate and power elite class that benefits from capitalism, to believe in an outcome that could never be possible, for the majority, but which supports the power and positions and wealth of that corporate and power elite class.

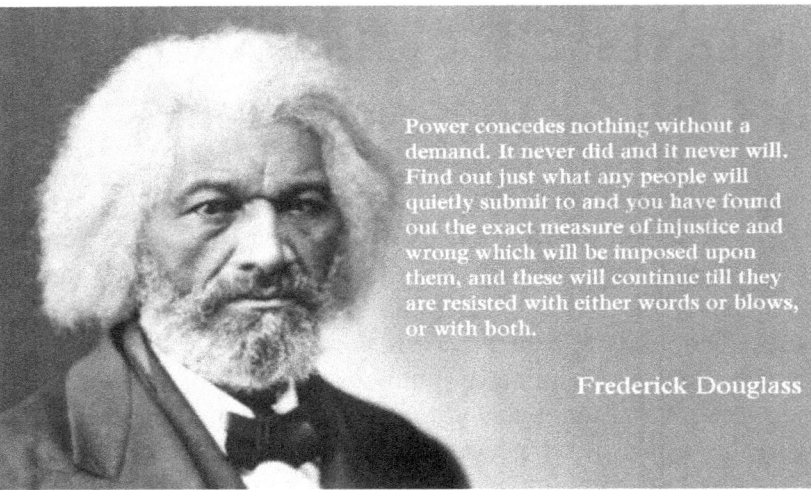

Power concedes nothing without a demand. It never did and it never will. Find out just what any people will quietly submit to and you have found out the exact measure of injustice and wrong which will be imposed upon them, and these will continue till they are resisted with either words or blows, or with both.

Frederick Douglass

Capitalism is not broken and never was; it is by design an economic structure that enriches the minority at the expense of the majority that ***must***, in the end, lead to the destruction of society by corrupting culture and politics and by subverting the public good in favor of the needs and desires of the capitalist power elite capitalists. This exploitation occurs, while convincing those that suffer under and or do not benefit from capitalism, through propaganda and censorship, which it is the best of all economic systems and that if they fail it is their fault and not the fault of the system. Therefore, it is working as designed and not as its apologists lament that we do not have capitalism but crony capitalism instead. They do not realize that <u>capitalism must lead to cronyism, fascism, kakistocracy[149], and corruption of social values, monopoly of wealth and power, and destruction of society</u> by its hoarding of wealth and rapacious greed that sacrifices all (human life and natural resources) on the altar of more wealth and power gain. These flaws of capitalism are not errors or anomalies but endemic features of that system of economic practice. Capitalism naturally and progressively allows greater participation of those afflicted by desire for and practice of rapacious greed, sociopaths and psychopaths to take up leadership positions where they are able to implement seemingly irrational but intentional policies that increase their wealth and power but lead to the subversion of social and political as well as economic institutions in favor of corruption, and untruths that sabotage the capacity of a society to live by facts, ethics and sound decision-making that promotes and sustains life. Instead, the delusions

---

[149] A **kakistocracy** (/kækɪˈstɒkrəsi/, /kækɪsˈtɒkrəsi/) is a system of government that is run by the worst, least qualified, and/or most unscrupulous citizens. The word was coined as early as the seventeenth century.

foisted by the sociopathic and psychopathic political and corporate (fascist) leaders produce collective social delusions that promote the death of society through the insanity of stress, pollution, conflict, and war. The collective social delusions see progress in pollution, more disease and political insanity, such as that demonstrated in the case of Donald Trump (intense narcissistic personality disorder) or the new president, Biden, who displays signs of senility, dementia and or alzheimer's disease).

The history of supposedly democratic countries (Europe, USA, Canada in particular) leading up to **the year 2020 demonstrated** that the societies were already, and had been for decades, entrenched in neoliberal policies and actions including barbarous empire-building, mass surveillance, disempowering the middle class and workers, and toppling governments worldwide so as to favor corporations and consolidate power under the USA empire.

The year 2020 revealed that the neoliberal agenda foisted on world populations was brought home to the peoples of those supposedly democratic countries, thus revealing those supposed democracies as shams; in other words, the veneer of democratic government is a façade hiding a fascistic rapacious ruthless and sociopathic power elite who are willing to implement policies up to and including murder, to achieve their goals of economic and political domination. An example of the willingness to achieve the goals of power and wealth is evident in the willingness to allow more deaths from their policies than would have occurred naturally with the coronavirus. There have been more suicides, more disease and more deaths from the policies of mask mandates, social distancing and lockdown policies than would have occurred if those policies had not been implemented. It is estimated that upwards of 85% of the deaths that occurred could have been avoided if they would have instead used known early treatments with supplements and safe drugs to treat the "coronavirus" or "covid 19" disease. Nevertheless, the safe supplements and drugs were discouraged and the policies were and continue to be promoted even as evidence continues to confirm the falsehoods about the claims that mask mandates, social distancing, lockdown policies, and unproven drugs and experimental vaccines are effective policies.

Tens of Thousands of Lives Could Have Been Saved if Research on COVID Treatments Hadn't Been Suppressed[150]

Fallacy of Crony Capitalism as a device allowing the power elite to appear in error, stupid or incompetent while in the end "stumbling" into enrichment and empire.

The year 2020 revealed the culmination of how capitalism developed over decades as the creeping power of the rich elite is used to bribe government authorities thereby corrupting politics, the judicial system, and all other substantial areas of the economy such as the media, the health industry, the land management, and food industries, banking and currency creation, police powers and tagging, tracing, monitoring through vaccines, expansion of smart devices with 5G and satellite surveillance. The Ancient Egyptian sage Amenemopet taught that luxuries are corruptions to the human character. That is because most humans take the path of least resistance and have a predilection for pleasure and convenience which corrupts ethics. Therefore, of course, these innovations, of modern society, touted as conveniences and luxuries of modern material culture, become dependencies not unlike drug addictions. Thus, in reality, those dependencies debilitate, erode and corrupt human conscience and ethical culture. They would not be possible without the willing support of the population that falls into the confidence game of modern conveniences, which degrade the personality and result in the addiction to pleasure-seeking through the luxury of conveniences, amenities, expediencies, and disdain for inconveniences. This degradation forces intellectual atrophy and weakened will. A prime example of crony fascist capitalism manifesting is the presidency of George W. Bush. He was regarded as a not bright person and as a bumbling, stumbling mentally challenged person. Yet his actions duped the nation into wars that served the goals of rapacious capitalists, war mongers and political neo-conservatives seeking world domination. His war crimes were never prosecuted and the country benefited from his and his political allies' actions, which included approval of torture and led to the

---

[150] https://stuartbramhall.wordpress.com/2021/05/13/tens-of-thousands-of-lives-could-have-been-saved-if-research-on-covid-treatments-hadnt-been-suppressed/
https://youtu.be/lL6U31QKOQc

deaths of thousands of soldiers and as many as 1 million persons in the other countries where the war machine was directed.

The year 2020 revealed, if it was not obvious previously, how the process of applying policies that seem rational or irrational that work out as errors or wrong policies, sometimes with "unintended" effects demonstrated that those aspects of the economy and the government are not "broken", as many people like to lament. Rather, these developments are natural and necessary processes in the development of fascist government and capitalism. The imposition of the seemingly irrational or wrong government policies is easy in the environment of a representative government system designed to facilitate power elite corruption policies with impunity. In other words, the government system itself is designed for empowering an oligarchy and disempowering the masses; so in reality, government is an arm of capitalism -in other words, there has been fascism all along, in varied degrees. Secondly, there is no such thing as capitalism as a benign force for good in the world or a system for producing wealth and benefit for society and the world. Capitalism, the accumulation of wealth (capital) in the hands of few power elite personalities and the control that it affords them over a society, corrupts the social, political and economic culture of a society. ***Therefore, capitalism must necessarily flower into fascism, the police state, surveillance state, tyranny, and totalitarianism.***

So, the choice is not between having good capitalism or bad capitalism or ethical capitalism or crony capitalism. In other words, the designs and ultimate objectives of capitalism are empire and fascism even as they may seem to begin benignly but in the end, nevertheless, the goal of capitalism is fascism and barbarous empire. This is what ultimately happens when this form of economics is allowed to take hold in a society. Therefore, there is no such thing as benevolent, good, or manageable capitalism. ALL capitalism leads to fascism, totalitarianism, and barbarianism in the end, even if it may take a few generations for the decay in social ethics, government ethics, and judicial ethics to fully degrade to a state where capitalism is able to emerge into its flowering rapacious fulminant, malignant form (fascist totalitarian police state). One of the reasons that capitalism is able to be so damaging to society is that it will always be the abode of that element of the population that is most capable of ruthlessness and callous disregard for human life and which will be willing to do whatever is necessary to achieve its goals even if that means their own death and or the death of their own country, society or family members. This is in reality the psychological pathology that a society opens itself up to when allowing capitalism (unbridled greed and lust for power) to take hold as its primary economic system. This is a psychological pathology, that in the end, leads to social self-destruction. The same outcome would occur in any similar type of government and economic systems, be they managed by supposed left-wingers such as communists or right-wingers such as conservative republicans. So the choice is not between political parties or economic ideologies but between an ethical government that supports ethical conscience based on universally agreed facts and evidence of what works and what promotes health and well-being for individuals and the society as a whole and protects the inalienable human and spiritual rights of people, their personal sovereignty, over the designs of sociopaths and psychopaths, their corporations or systems that promote the opportunity of those sociopaths and psychopaths to gain control of society, corrupt its discourse, ethics, politics, and economics for their own benefit and the detriment of everyone else.

USA GOVERNMENT DESIGNED FOR TYRANNY OF THE MINORITY OVER THE MAJORITY.

The system of government used in the USA is not democracy and never was intended to be "democratic". This is the reasoning behind the quote by Benjamin Franklin. Pure democracy facilitates the tyranny of a majority over a minority. That discovery was made back in the classical Greek period when democracy was invented, as its application was easily manipulated by the leaders. Therefore, by definition, democracy, as a governing system, cannot produce a fair and ethical government. However, neither can the representative form of government lead to prosperity, equality, sanity and ethics. Representative government produces a façade of democracy but in reality empowers an oligarchy that employs capitalism and fascism to exploit the society, in other words, a kakistocracy. In essence, the American Revolution replaced a rapacious feudal monarchy system with a rapacious oligarchic capitalist system. The so-called founding fathers of the USA knew about this flaw of democracy and steered away from giving power to people directly, but they gave the power to themselves, the oligarchs/aristocrats. Hence the creation of several tiers of government bodies separating the ordinary citizen from the true levers of governmental power. The USA has the reverse, a system that fools people into thinking they have democratic input when in reality it is a system that facilitates the tyranny of the minority over the majority.

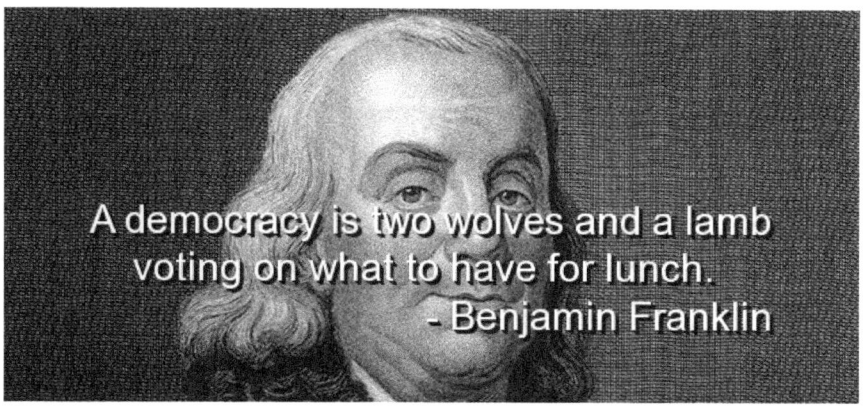

One of the most important obstacles to having righteous government, politics, and economics is the fall, by the members of society, into the slippery slope of reductionist thinking and belief that there is a given political/economic ideology or ideologically correct political party that is better than any others, that holds their concerns at heart and that those concerns, being correct, lead to prosperity and they have the right to impose that on others, even against their will or over their personal sovereignty. Such a belief system holds that if others disagree then they are wrong and should be disempowered and not negotiated with for the greater good of all. This kind of orthodoxy, which believes itself to be the only source of "truth" and consequently the sole purveyor of "truth", is usually seen in many fundamentalist religions, but also manifests in the government and the social mind of the public, in the form of political religious fundamentalism operating as subconscious motivations that sustain unethical and unjust as well as irrational, ideological beliefs and policies. This is all fueled by the blind-faith in the political party and sustained by the personal degradations described earlier; some due to endemic flaws in the human personality and others fomented or exploited by the sociopathic leaders. Democracy, though it is touted by government elites in most modern cultures as a process promoting freedom and the public good, is, in reality, a mechanism to create an artifice of public will (manufacturing consent[151]) that is, in reality, a manipulated public opinion that serves no legislative purpose except to rubber-stamp the power elite policies, since the will of the electorate has almost no effect[152] on the policies of the government officials as they are to some degree, all controlled by corporations and the power elites.

---

[151] MANUFACTURING CONSENT: THE POLITICAL ECONOMY OF THE MASS MEDIA by Edward S. Herman and Noam Chomsky | Jan 15, 2002
[152] PRINCETON STUDY: U.S. NO LONGER AN ACTUAL DEMOCRACY- APRIL 18, 2014
https://talkingpointsmemo.com/livewire/princeton-experts-say-us-no-longer-democracy

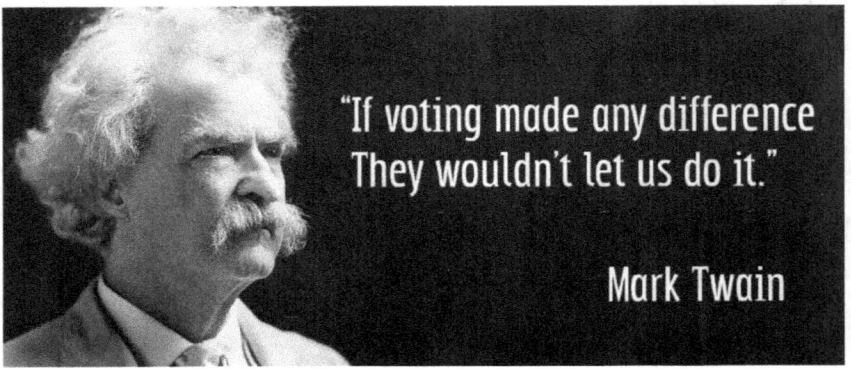

"We have one country, one Constitution and one future that binds us."
-president George W. Bush

"Stop throwing the Constitution in my face," Bush screamed back. "It's just a goddamned piece of paper!"[153]
-President George W. Bush

> Those who vote decide nothing.
>
> Those who count the vote decide everything.
>
> -- Joseph Stalin

The duplicity of former president G. W. Bush belies the fraud of political rhetoric that seems to speak of a common honest intent to live by constitutionally agreed principles but that in reality seeks to subvert those principles even as it portrays itself as their champion. The aforesaid degraded perspective operates in the devolved society and that degraded state is ripe for political demagogues and manipulations by the power elite. The duplicity of presidents is aided and abetted by political machiavellians, who operate on behalf of the power

---

[153] https://rense.com/general69/paper.htm

elites, such as Henry Kissinger, who more directly and openly carry out the nefarious, illegal, and immoral acts of despotism, subversion, and empire-building both at home and abroad. An example of a machiavellian technocrat, doing the bidding of the political machiavellian, on behalf of the power elites, is William Casey, CIA Director.

> **"The illegal we do immediately; the unconstitutional takes a little longer."**
>
> **"Depopulation should be the highest priority of foreign policy towards the third world."**
>
> -Henry Kissinger

========

> Turns out I'm really good at killing people,"
> -president Barak Obama
>
> The quote comes in the context of both the drone program and the killing of Osama bin Laden by a special forces strike force. The passage also specifically references the death of another al Qaeda leader, Anwar al-Awlaki, who was killed by a CIA drone strike in Yemen on Sept. 30, 2011.[154]

We may ask why is it that after hearing Obama's own assessment of himself as a "killer", people would still reelect him in overwhelming numbers? In particular, many African-Americans voted for him simply because he seemed to be African American like them. Many "white" people voted for Mitt Romney simply because he was "white". From the perspective of the masses, their votes were based on identity politics and racism and not on ethical considerations, like evidence of competency, sanity, honesty, track record of service to humanity, etc. From the perspective of the power elites, they did not care which one would win since either would follow their dictates or be maneuvered into the power elite policies through control of banking, Wall Street and the media. When does unrestricted killing become a permissible act by a government official? When did the moral outrage of the idea of a person, be it king or president, having the ability to kill with impunity erode to the point of apathy? Wasn't this issue a supposed primary factor sparking the American revolution and the subsequent US constitution? This issue, as described about Obama, who did little if

---

[154] https://www.huffpost.com/entry/obama-drones-double-down_n_4208815

anything for the African American community, was no different than many people who identify themselves as "white" or European-Americans, voted for those candidates who seem to resemble them even though the elected persons prove they do not have the interests of the public at heart. This points to the inability or unwillingness of the general population to live by ethical principles and instead participate willingly in or fall prey to the frauds perpetrated by sociopaths and criminals. Thus, the members of the public are also complicit in the pathologies, delusions, and criminality of their leaders by following their dictates, without question, and not voting for those who demonstrate higher ethics; in reality, voting for the lesser of two evils is not the answer; the answer is to change the systems of politics and economics to one based on ethics instead of supporting one based on corruption, cronyism, and identity politics.

There can be no fair and free democracy in an environment of flawed government systems coupled with corrupt, sociopathic, criminal leaders, mass surveillance, and political coercion. However, fair and ethical government also cannot exist in an environment of selfishness, greed, hatred, fear, and deep-seated anxieties in the populace. In other words, the concept of democracy is bound to fail because it is flawed, and also normal humans are susceptible to corruption. Even if the stated purpose of the so-called "democratic government" is the production of a balanced and well-adjusted society, it will inevitably produce opportunities for the human wolves (con artists, sociopaths, and psychopaths) to take advantage of the sheep, the ignorant, immature, neurotic, flawed members of society and commit atrocities that will be even supported by some of those same members of society who are susceptible to party ideologies, greed, fears, etc. (sheeple[155]). This very situation is what, as proven by the *Princeton Study*[156], the US political landscape has become; a society in which the politics, which were never a democracy, to begin with (the USA government was set up as a constitutional republic managed by aristocrat landowners) has descended to outright and open plutocracy.[157] The failure of the masses to realize this fact allows the plutocracy[158] class, which is

---

[155] People who are meekly submissive or easily swayed.
[156] PRINCETON STUDY: U.S. NO LONGER AN ACTUAL DEMOCRACY- APRIL 18, 2014
https://talkingpointsmemo.com/livewire/princeton-experts-say-us-no-longer-democracy
[157] IBID
[158] A plutocracy (Greek: πλοῦτος, ploutos, 'wealth' + κράτος, kratos, 'power') or plutarchy is a society that is ruled or controlled by people of great wealth or income. The first known use of the term in English dates from 1631.

composed of an oligarchy[159] of elites to rule with impunity over the whole society. This is the reason why the political satirist and comedian, George Carlin, referred to the "American Dream" as something one must be asleep to be believing in; meaning that people are socially and politically asleep (corrupted morals, corrupted ethics, deluded by promises of wealth and security by the power elite politicians and media, reinforced by other deluded people and family that have fallen for the confidence-game (swindle/fraud/scam/rip-off/embezzlement/racket/theft) called the "American Dream".[160]

THE PURPOSEFUL FAILURE OF TRICKLE-DOWN ECONOMICS, LOWER INTEREST RATES, AND BAIL-OUTS THAT ENRICH THE POWER ELITES AND IMPOVERISH EVERYONE ELSE.

The economic strategy of bailing out corporations and lowering interest rates, supposedly to save the economy, has for years proven to be a failure in terms of being a solution to the underlying financial problems of income and wealth inequality. It has been a failure just as the "trickledown theory", begun during the Reagan presidency years, has been proven to be false. Instead of money trickling down the economy to the common person, more of the money and wealth stays with the rich. The strategy of bailouts and lowering interest rates, supposedly to spur the economy and stave off deflation, actually causes inflation and also deflation for the population and enrichment of the rich and power elite by their having access to the newly created bailout currency funds (Cantillon Effect) and the capacity to use cheap or free currency funds to buy off politicians, create monopolies, control the economy and purchase assets cheaply while the common person lives on subsistence wages or welfare[161] in an environment of ever-rising consumer prices. Therefore, the history of the last 40 years has demonstrated that the financial strategies imposed by the central banks are actually self-serving strategies that enrich the rich and impoverish the middle and lower class instead of enriching all members of the economy. Under capitalism, there can be no such thing as a "free market" because the

---

[159] **Oligarchy** (from Greek ὀλιγαρχία *(oligarkhía)*; from ὀλίγος *(olígos)* 'few', and ἄρχω *(arkho)* 'to rule or to command') is a form of power structure in which power rests with a small number of people. These people may be distinguished by nobility, wealth, education, corporate, religious, political, or military control. Such states are often controlled by families who pass their influence from one generation to the next, but inheritance is not a necessary condition of oligarchy.
[160] The real owners are the big wealthy business interests that control things and make
[161] https://www.youtube.com/watch?v=EoJxPaJ6nu0

people with means in the form of capital will move to corrupt the markets in their favor directly or by bribing politicians to make laws in their favor. Thus, by definition, capitalism includes manipulated, corrupted markets to benefit those doing the corruptions. Therefore, "free market capitalism" is a pipe dream and instead the term "free market capitalism" should be thought of as an Orwellian euphemism or propaganda meme tool that has the opposite meaning. That tool is used by those who are not aware of the fraudulent self-serving purpose of the "free markets" which is to defraud the population and enrich the few capitalists, the power elite.

> "The conscious and intelligent manipulation of the organized habits and opinions of the masses is an important element in democratic society. Those who manipulate this unseen mechanism of society constitute an invisible government which is the true ruling power of our country. ...We are governed, our minds are molded, our tastes formed, our ideas suggested, largely by men we have never heard of. This is a logical result of the way in which our democratic society is organized. Vast numbers of human beings must cooperate in this manner if they are to live together as a smoothly functioning society. ...In almost every act of our daily lives, whether in the sphere of politics or business, in our social conduct or our ethical thinking, we are dominated by the relatively small number of persons...who understand the mental processes and social patterns of the masses. It is they who pull the wires which control the public mind."
> — Edward Bernays, Propaganda

The delusions about USA capitalism and supposed democracy, about how it is fundamentally good and is not an instrument of social delusion and not an empire that commits war crimes and toppling governments and does not collude with corporations to impoverish its own people, along with the delusion that it only needs to be reformed somehow or that everything is fine with it if we get rid of a "few" wrong, bad apples, but they are not sociopathic, persons, etc.; these delusions, perpetrated by the corporations, the media and power elites, constitute a serious and fatal vulnerability in the mind of the populace that serves the purpose of oligarchy and social control by the power elites and corrupt corporations. Therefore, "American Democracy" is a front for violent, rapacious capitalism, exploitation, and enslavement as well as sociopathic tyrannical totalitarianism just as corrupted socialist governments, of the past, such as the Nazi government of mid-20th century Germany. The delusion about democracy and the American dream serves as an ideology that comforts the pathological need for safety and security and prosperity in both the democratic and republican party followers. This pathology, that operates within liberals as well as conservatives, seeks out media echo chambers, available in either in-person or online social media interactions, in which it can repeatedly hear only messages that are supportive rhetoric that confirms the delusion and excludes dissenting ideas or proofs about the flaws or fallacies of those delusions. The echo chamber venues (partisan ideological online, talk radio, and TV cable news programs) reinforce and exacerbate the delusions leading to toxic social interactions that guide people to irrationality, mob mentality, hatred, intolerance, fear, and violence. As Edward Bernays said, this is all orchestrated and managed by the elites. Thus, the current pathology within the populace, that supports the toxic social media environment, along with the politics and economics are used to confuse and pit groups against each other by exacerbating fears and ignorance. Under these conditions, the existential crisis of global warming/climate change, will not be faced and whatever happens will be based on the decisions of the power elite, which show predilection towards control and policies that promote continued exploitation at the cost of environmental disaster and medical atrocities caused by rapacious pharmaceutical industry[162] treatments, such as promoting chemical gene therapies under the guise of vaccines instead of promoting known lifesaving medicines and nutritional supplements that have been shown to actually save lives. The power elite, operating through central banks, corporations and bought off government officials, have no interest in changing polluting industries and commerce or changing the economic system from capitalism and profit at any cost, to sustainable economics that promotes life and health, environmental protection along with ethical distribution of resources, as those changes do not benefit their power and wealth interests.

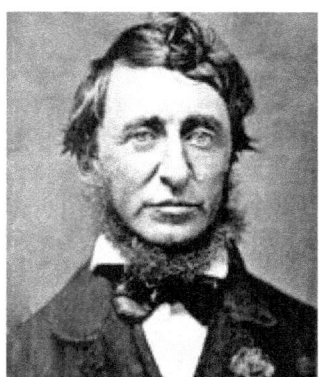

"The preachers and lecturers deal with men of straw, as they are men of straw themselves. Why, a free-spoken man, of sound lungs, cannot draw a long breath without causing your rotten institutions to come toppling down by the vacuum he makes. Your church is a baby-house

---

[162] https://garynull.com/another-chapter-in-history-of-irresponsible-medical-practice/

made of blocks,[163] and so of the state.

>...The church, the state, the school, the magazine, think they are liberal and free! It is the freedom of a prison-yard."
> — Henry David Thoreau[164]

The fallacy that most people are living under, that their country is better than others and that they are free or that one party is better than another or that one person, gender, or color is better than another was displayed as the democrats won the election in Nov. 2020. In 2008 when a "black" man, Obama and the democratic party won, many people thought that real change would come to the country while others went out to buy guns, thinking the democrats want to disarm them. The republican party operatives did not dissuade their followers in their unfounded beliefs and immediately set out to thwart any political agenda he might have campaigned on. Obama did not disarm anyone but instead started several new wars including the destruction of one country, Libya. So, that 2008 election, won by Obama, was dreaded by those who are in the republican party or otherwise oppose the neoliberal agenda. In 2016 the win by Trump was dreaded by the democrats and they immediately set out to discredit him by propagandizing a hoax that he was a Russian "agent". In all the cases above, the ordinary voters, the followers of the political parties, followed in lockstep, (ideologically, not ethically) believing the ideological rhetoric of their party leaders, without exercising critical thinking about the worth of the candidates or the lies that were spread on each side about the other. In this same way, people are also following the lies not only from the political parties and the media but also from the supposed medical "authorities".

The aforesaid highlights the danger of living in an unethical society based on political ideologies and identity politics instead of righteousness and truth based on ethics and verifiable facts. It also points out the danger of living in a society where people do not act out of thoughtful consideration followed by emotional expression but rather the reverse. They act first out of feelings and emotions followed by thoughtless (stunted intellect) rationalized reactions. At worse, due to fear, they act out of animal instinct, having been miseducated, and conditioned by propaganda.

---

[163] Similar concept as "house of cards"
[164] I to Myself: An Annotated Selection from the Journal of Henry D. Thoreau

Although he was maneuvered, by the power elites, into bombing Syria, Trump, at least appeared to have tried to not escalate aggression against the country Syria. Unlike Trump and like Obama, in early 2021 the new president Biden took over and immediately mobilized US armed forces to go back into one of the countries invaded by Obama, Syria. Biden additionally brought back into his administration most of the lobbyists and political operatives that worked under him and Obama, making sure the corporations have a voice in the policies, signaling that the same corruption, foreign policy, and domestic agenda of exploitation and enriching corporations would be affirmed. The aforesaid points to the delusion that most people are under, that the republicans are warmongers and corporate supporters and the democrats are the peacemakers and financial supporters of the "people". Thus, both the political parties, in the USA, represent the same support of empire and the designs of the power elite, only from apparent superficially polar opposite standpoints; while they may differ on social issues, substantively they support the same agenda of domestic and international domination and exploitation. This means that it is foolish to seek refuge in or justice from a political system based on rapacious greed, power, and control that has demonstrated willingness to apply tyranny to the international and domestic populations on behalf of corporations and the power elite. Also, there can be no righteous, just government when people cede their rights to sociopathic leaders and follow them out of fear or ignorance and are not able to take part (due to personal compromised ethics, political electoral frauds and corporate media propaganda and censorship, all in an environment of surveillance and capitalist financial coercion and fear due to their capacity to provide or withdraw jobs from the public) in the legislative process and are not able to submit political corporate leaders to strict ethical and legal penalties. In the first month of his presidency, the new president, wasted no time in returning to the neoliberal imperial warmongering policies of his democrat party predecessor, Obama.

Biden says he told foreign leaders "America is back"
-President Joe Biden January 2021

Just Like the Good Old Days: Joe Biden Invades Syria with Convoy of US Troops and Choppers on First Full Day as President

-news report January 23, 202

The degraded state of affairs, in the year 2020, culminated in the supposed victory of the democrats in the elections held in November, under a cloud of apparent election fraud, just as previous year's elections had been under the same cloud when republicans had won the elections (election fraud on both sides). The mistrust of the media and fear about losing Donald Trump, a person supported perhaps not for his cultured or ethical personality or any real benefit to the common person during his presidency, but because for some, he was an outlet for the nativist, racist, or misogynist, feelings and the need for a father authority figure (due to the fears instilled in the population). The racist issues had at least two dimensions; one the fear of white men of losing their livelihood and social standing in society and another, the irrational learned fear, mistrust, and hatred of those who are not "white". For some, he represented a shield protecting gun rights and by extension an ideal of liberty against the tyranny of government. For others, he apparently represented a protest against the Democratic Party and Republican Party corruptions and was supported because there was no other alternative way to make such a protest vote.

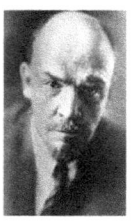

"The Capitalists will sell us the rope with which we will hang them."
~ Vladimir Ilyich Lenin

The threat of the USA government and power elite to its own population may only be surpassed by the threat of its USA metastasized creation in the form of the Chinese communist government capitalism system. In the early 1970s the USA government and corporations (fascism-headed by the Western Power elites) entered into a plan, partly directed at turning China away from the Power elites headed by Russia (at the time USSR) to help China industrialize so as to benefit from their cheap labor. In doing so the communist party, composed of the oligarchic power elite global predator class, of that country, was able to receive the capital investment, expertise, and technological capability of the USA and other western countries, which was, again, given, by USA and other western countries, willingly.

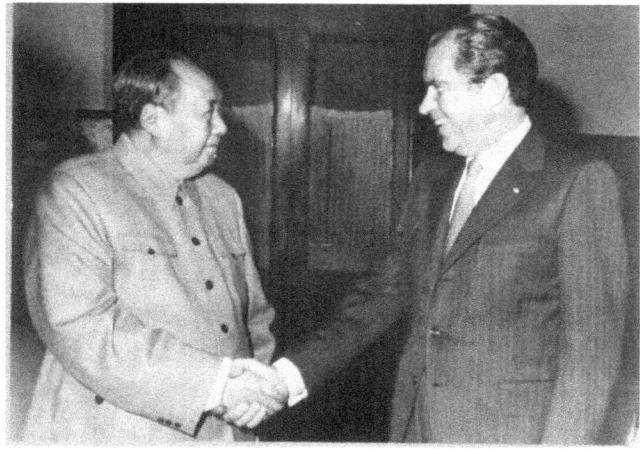

USA president Nixon shakes hands with Chinese leader Mao Zedong (1972)

Beginning in the early 1970s' the Chinese used the capital investment, expertise, and technological capability of the USA (which the USA corporations willingly, out of greed, gave to the Chinese, with the blessing of republican and democrat politicians-hence the statement by Lenin) to create an industrial base that is surpassing the USA and empowered the first full totalitarian surveillance fascistic police state in China. Now, in 2020-2021 the USA and other western countries are trying to follow the example of China's surveillance police state fascistic control (vaccine passport and social credit scheme) over its population especially in the wake of the fraudulent coronavirus pandemic as an excuse for the need to have more surveillance, tracking and the institution of currency controls (currency great reset). The Chinese government is using its power to buy up resources around the world and undermine local institutions of other countries including the USA to favor their policies and designs which involve megalomaniacal world domination. Unlike previous empires, which tried to dominate by force of arms, this empire is doing so through business arrangements and the tried and true method of buying off local officials and additionally also digitally controlling public opinion through propaganda and censorship. Thus, China now has developed into a fascistic totalitarian communist government with a capitalist economic system while the USA has a fascistic totalitarian representative republic government with a capitalist economy. Just as the USA did spread globalization and western capitalism and its brand of fascism, and military CIA subversive neo-colonialism around the world, so too China is moving ahead to spread its brand of eastern capitalism now with social credit scores, surveillance subversive financial neo-colonialism. In the western countries, social credit scores will first take the form of "vaccine passports" and then the control mechanisms pioneered by China will be incorporated into the *vaccine passport digital surveillance police state model*. The two-factor total totalitarian control and absolute loss of individual freedoms will be complete when the *central bank digital currency*[165] is fully implemented along with the vaccine passports.

China's social credit program creeps into Canada[166]

THE CORONAVIRUS AND THE GLOBAL PLAN OF DOMINATION BY THE POWER ELITES

The imposed lockdowns on societies worldwide were supposed to be temporary (2 weeks), to supposedly slow the progression of illness by "flattening the curve" of new infections. That never worked. As of the date of this writing (1 year and 3 months after their commencement), they have not been stopped, along with facemask wearing mandates that have been both proven ineffective; yet they are still being pushed by supposed health authorities including CDC, without scientific evidence. Since peer-reviewed science has, many months ago, verified that there is no medical or social benefit of mask-wearing, social distancing, and

---

[165] https://www.corbettreport.com/interview-1604-john-titus-on-central-bank-digital-currencies/
https://www.youtube.com/watch?v=yI3rmlgw20s
https://www.youtube.com/watch?v=UOxvjhd2HJw
[166] https://www.sundayguardianlive.com/news/chinas-social-credit-program-creeps-canada

lockdowns we are left with the conclusion that it is being done for other purposes, such as training and eliciting compliance and
submission to the government, the impoverishment of the population and forced dependency on government handouts for subsistence-level existence. This also has the effect of impoverishing political activism and support for populist candidates that criticize or oppose the current system of government, which has, for decades, been steadily moving towards fascism (working with and in support of corporations and the impoverishment of the masses). The centralization impoverishes the masses while forcing their financial weakness in a hierarchical form of top-down control that supersedes individual governments.

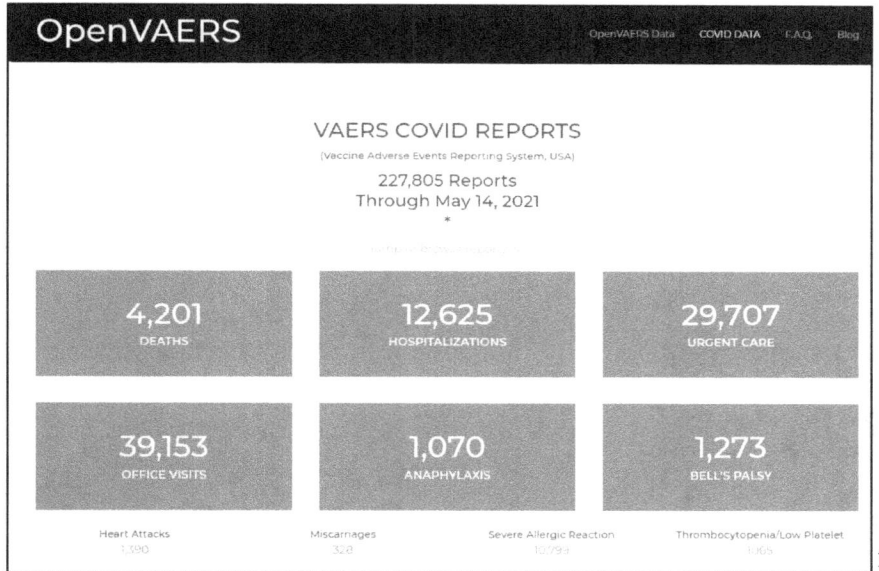

[167][168]

Note: the figures above are estimated to be only between 1%-10% of the real total. So these figures are low estimates.

As of the date (May 2021) the new so-called untested, unproven, and therefore unsafe chemicals, they have labeled as "vaccines", are being administered and as a direct result over 4000[169] people have died along with

---

[167] https://www.openvaers.com/covid-data
https://www.medalerts.org/vaersdb/findfield.php?EVENTS=on&PAGENO=1&PERPAGE=10&ESORT&REVERSESORT&VAX=%28COVID19%29&VAXTYPES=%28COVID-19%29&DIED=Yes&fbclid=IwAR2rBWzmzUUh-5eWc3N4gp6PV3aEnpIyzAX0Oazu32g8hzrPHqKfVmflV1M
[168] ibid
[169] covid data (it is estimated that only 1% of vaccine adverse events is reported)

tens of thousands of injuries due to severe reactions.[170] The now international, coordinated policy displaying the willingness to enforce face masks and lockdowns, that have been proven to be more harmful and deadly, killing more people than the supposed virus, leading to depression, financial lives destroyed, suicides, domestic and child abuse, etc.[171] points to the now not farfetched conspiracy theory that there is a power elites global agenda. That global agenda is now an open, stated strategy, by the members of the "world economic forum", that sees the coronavirus as an "opportunity" to change society. The changes include moving from physical to digital currency, rental instead of ownership, no privacy through digital surveillance including tagging everyone and reduction of the population. Thus, they have also publicly announced that the coronavirus is an "opportunity" to facilitate the pursuit of their goals to accomplish a financial "great reset" that will transform capitalism into what is essentially a neo-feudal system of politics and economics in which people will supposedly "own nothing and be happy". These goals are to be achieved under the guise of working towards supposed vague concepts, that sound desirable, such as "inclusivity" and tackling the global warming issue, wherein the power elite would be, of course, included in the ownership class that would control everything in society.

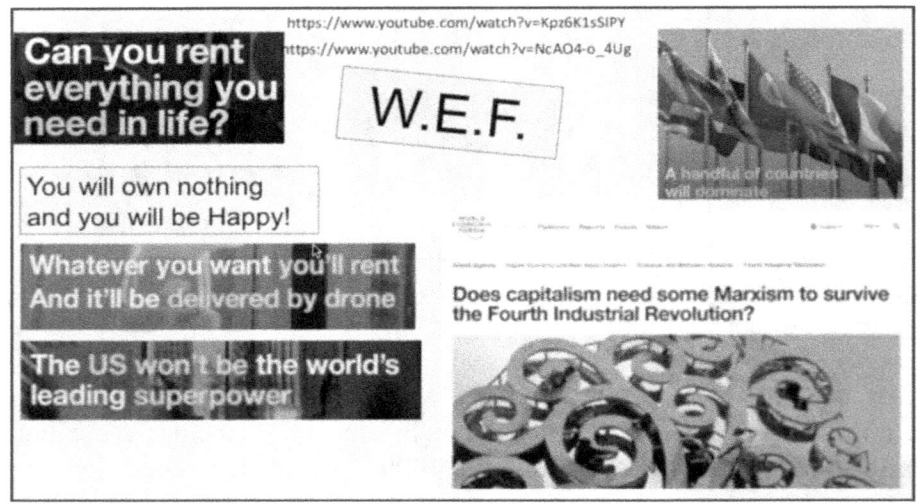

[170] https://www.medalerts.org/vaersdb/findfield.php?EVENTS=on&PAGENO=1&PERPAGE=10&ESORT&REVERSESORT&VAX=%28COVID19%29&VAXTYPES=%28COVID-19%29&DIED=Yes&fbclid=IwAR2rBWzmzUUh-5eWc3N4gp6PV3aEnpIyzAX0Oazu32g8hzrPHqKfVmflV1M

[171] THE NEW GREAT DEPRESSION: WINNERS AND LOSERS IN A POST-PANDEMIC WORLD HARDCOVER – JANUARY 12, 2021
by James Rickards

> **WORLD ECONOMIC FORUM**
> https://www.weforum.org/agenda/2020/07/to-build-back-better-we-must-reinvent-capitalism-heres-how
>
> **To build back better, we must reinvent capitalism. Here's how**
>
> Thanks to the ongoing pandemic, the world is off-balance – and it will remain so for years to come. Far from settling into a 'new normal', we should expect a COVID-19 domino effect, triggering further disruptions – positive as well as negative – over the decade ahead.
>
> The wave of civil unrest that spread across America and beyond recently may be one example; it seems likely that the pandemic contributed to the context in which anger and despair boiled over into outrage and unrest following the death of George Floyd.
>
> Other possible COVID-induced discontinuities ahead range from a full-blown financial crisis to a step change in the rate of the global energy transition: some analysts now reckon **that fossil fuel demand may have peaked in 2019 – for good.**
> The virus has highlighted **many vulnerabilities – within businesses, supply chains, economies, health systems and political institutions – that will need to be addressed in the post-crisis world.** It has underscored the interconnectedness of our natural, social and economic systems, and provided a stark reminder of the scale of systemic risks that can build up when we allow weaknesses and negative impacts to accumulate over time.

An interesting correlation was pointed out, by documentary filmmaker Claudia Nye, about the countries where the supposed new virus initially hit first. It turns out that the G20 countries were affected first.[172] The virus affected those countries first and the imposition of irrational, contradictory regulations including the forcing of businesses to close down in response, caused major economic damage in those countries. The economic devastation that was experienced in countries that imposed the, on the surface, apparently irrational and useless measures to "combat" coronavirus was not experienced in countries such as Sweden, which did not impose mask-wearing, social distancing, and lockdowns. Seeing the now well-known examples of Sweden, as well as the examples of other countries, such as Japan, Taiwan, countries in Africa and states in the USA[173] that did not impose those measures and yet suffered less or no economic devastation AND less disease and deaths, while still promoting and imposing those failed regulations in the other G20 countries, signals an ulterior motivation. Many view the actions by officials, over the last year, as a purposeful strategy to allow the disease to take hold and proliferate in those areas but also to promote economic devastation wherein wealthy individuals and corporations can take advantage by acquiring those assets, from the bankrupted lower, middle and upper classes, at minimal cost and

---

[172] The **G20** (or **Group of Twenty**) is an international forum for the governments and central bank governors from 19 countries and the European Union (EU). They meet to "coordinate" world economic activity.
[173] https://usafacts.org/visualizations/coronavirus-covid-19-spread-map/
https://www.mercurynews.com/2020/11/10/these-are-the-15-states-that-dont-require-masks/

thereby become richer.[174] The result of developing increased disease and confusion in the population along with general stress, confusion, incapacity to hold meetings and protest government policies and economic devastation and promoting impoverishment are parts of the ulterior motives.

Along with the effect of impoverishing people with the lockdowns, the low interest rates and bailouts have the effect of lowering the value of all currencies even more than the devaluation that has occurred since the creation of the Federal Reserve bank and the fractional banking system with built-in inflation that robs the wealth of all users of the currency slowly over time. Currency is not money. Paper dollars or government decreed transaction notes are fiat, decreed currency with no real value. Those worth-less currency notes have been imposed on society by the power elites through the banking system. Gold is real money; hence the saying "he who has the gold makes the rules" and hence the desire of power elites to own gold and discourage others from owning gold. Inflation occurs when governments add currency to the current existing amount of currency. The new currency, for bailouts, was created out of thin air, not being based on any economic activity or wealth creation. It benefits the banks and corporations and devalues the currency already held by everyone else. General, endemic inflation is a slow and steady means of impoverishing the population. The use of social, political or medical crises to justify lower interest rates, bailouts and currency creation to give to corporations and banks is an accelerated devaluation and consequently accelerated impoverishment of the population and accelerated enrichment of the moneyed class. The influential investor **Warren Buffet** and the influential economist, **John Maynard Keynes,** wrote about inflation honestly, as a forced tax on the population that impoverishes them, listing its undermining and devastating consequences. In 1977 the investor Warren Buffet referred to inflation as "inflation tax."

---

[174]https://articles.mercola.com/sites/articles/archive/2021/02/11/lockdown.aspx?ui=152220df1deda081f73727bc10a8407027b248ba493a7ce71f4a1e73a6c1d882&sd=20200829&cid_source=dnl&cid_medium=email&cid_content=art1HL&cid=20210211&mid=DM801843&rid=1081645302
https://youtu.be/Ri_yU_gHLcA

The writer Thomas M. Humphrey detailed Keyne's views on inflation:

> "By a continuing process of inflation, governments can confiscate, secretly and unobserved, an important part of the wealth of their citizens. There is no subtler, no surer means of overturning the existing basis of society than to debauch the currency. The process engages all the hidden forces of economic law on the side of destruction, and does it in a manner which not one man in a million is able to diagnose."
>
> ~ John Maynard Keynes
> (1883-1946) British economist
> "The Economic Consequences Of The Peace"

Early Writings

Keynes' strong aversion to inflation is evident in even his earliest work. It appears, for example, in his *Indian Currency and Finance* (1913). There he emphatically rejects the argument that "a depreciating currency is advantageous . . . to trade," contending that any advantages derived from inflation are "only temporary" and that they "occur largely at the expense of other members of the community" and therefore do "not profit the country as a whole" [5; p. 2]. He takes an even tougher attitude in his *Economic Consequences of the Peace* (1919), condemning inflation in the harshest possible terms. He says:

> Lenin is said to have declared that the best way to destroy the capitalist system was to debauch the currency. By a continuing process of inflation, governments can confiscate, secretly and unobserved, an important part of the wealth of their citizens. By this method they not only confiscate, but they confiscate arbitrarily; and, while the process impoverishes many, it actually enriches some [6; pp. 148-9].

He agrees with Lenin that inflation has the potentiality of destroying the basis of capitalist society.

> Lenin was certainly right. There is no subtler, no surer means of overturning the existing basis of society than to debauch the currency. The process engages all the hidden forces of economic law on the side of destruction, and does it in a manner which not one man in a million is able to diagnose [6; p. 149].

He then proceeds to specify at least four ways that rapid inflation works to weaken the social fabric and to undermine the foundations of the capitalist free-market system. First, unforeseen inflation, he says, results in a capricious and totally "arbitrary rearrangement of riches" that violates the principles of distributive justice. Besides its inequities, inflation also renders business undertakings riskier and thereby turns "the process of wealth-getting . . . into a gamble and a lottery." In generating risk and injustice, inflation "strikes not only at security, but at confidence in the equity of the existing distribution of wealth" [6; p. 149]. Second, inflation violates long-term arrangements based on the assumed stability of the value of money. In so doing, inflation disturbs contracts and upsets "all permanent relations between debtors and creditors, which form the ultimate foundation of capitalism" [6; p. 149]. Third, inflation generates social discontent and directs it against businessmen whose windfall profits are wrongly perceived to be the cause rather than the consequence of inflation. This discontent is exploited by governments which "being many of them . . . reckless . . . as well as weak, seek to direct on to a class known as 'profiteers' the popular indignation against the more obvious consequences of their vicious methods" [6; p. 149]. In other words, governments actually responsible for causing inflation seek to shift the blame onto businessmen who consequently lose "confidence in their place in society" and become "the easy victims of intimidation" by "governments of their own making,

and a Press of which they are the proprietors" [6; p. 150]. By making business a scapegoat and target of vilification and control, inflation reinforces anti-business attitudes and weakens support for what Keynes called "the active and constructive element in the whole capitalist society"[2] [6; p. 149].

Finally, inflation tends to breed such misguided remedies as "price regulation" and "profiteer-hunting" that may do more damage than the inflation itself. Keynes was especially critical of the tendency of governments to resort to price controls, which in his view lead to resource misallocation and a reduced supply of goods, thereby compounding inflationary pressures.[3] Regarding the disincentives to real output occasioned by controls, he said that "the preservation of a spurious value for the currency, by the force of law expressed in the regulation of prices, contains in itself, however, the seeds of final economic decay, and soon dries up the source of ultimate supply." For, by freezing prices at what are likely to be disequilibrium levels, controls constitute "a system of compelling the exchange of commodities at what is not their real relative value," and this "not only relaxes production but leads finally to the waste and inefficiency of barter" [6; pp. 149-50].

Summarizing the foregoing harmful consequences of inflation, he concludes that governments that allow inflation to get out of control do irreparable damage to the established social and economic order. In so doing they are "carrying a step further the fatal process which the subtle mind of Lenin had consciously conceived." For,

> By combining a popular hatred of the class of entrepreneurs with the blow already given to social security by the violent and arbitrary disturbance of contract and of the established equilibrium of wealth which is the inevitable result of inflation, these governments are fast rendering impossible a continuance of the social and economic order. . . . But they have no plan for replacing it [6; p. 150].

It would be difficult indeed to find a more damning indictment of inflation and inflationist policies than that presented by Keynes in *The Economic Consequences of the Peace*. Anyone seeking evidence that he was an inflationist will not find it there; on the contrary, not only does he display a marked aversion to inflation, but he also sees no compensating benefits to offset its evils.

The intention, of the banking system, under the direction of power elite personalities, is to use the currency to impoverish people by diminishing their wealth, through purposeful inflation of the currency, followed by purchasing assets with currency created by computer clicks on the bank computer accounts. So, under the central banking system, things that people have to work hard for in order to buy can be acquired by banks and their owners by simply counterfeiting the currency into existence – i.e. for free. This has the effect of enriching them (without their having to work to get the currency as others have to), controlling assets of real value, while the currency diminishes in value and eventually will be destroyed, at which time a digital currency will be introduced as a substitute wherein they will be able to digitally track[175] and control who gets currency by clicks on the same computer and have greater ability to steal the wealth of the users and also greater power to impose the police state. With the central bank digital currency anyone who opposes the power elites can be easily and instantly demonetized; anyone who purchases things that they do not want to be purchased can be stopped instantly; ability to transact financially, such as buying something at the corner store or fund transfers between countries can be instantly monitored and controlled, the ability to know where one is all the time can allow or disallow geographical movements and transactions. This is complete digital control. In short, it will be absolute financial control and the complete end of any semblance of financial or physical freedom. If further digitization is pursued, there is now the possibility of, through the technology that is currently available, of microchipping[176] to tag and monitor people and later monitor thoughts through trans-humanism, the possibility of monitoring thoughts and controlling people through digital impulses is not unforeseeable as these areas of research are currently being advanced.

In such a scenario, as described above, the world populations could be controlled by the power elite of the most powerful countries through technocrat personnel (ignorant, or immoral or amoral, deluded, government, police and military workers), the technocrats and blind followers or people living in fear and willing to submit for any handouts in order to survive. We have seen how certain personalities in police forces and the military are

---

[175] https://www.ft.com/content/88f47c48-97fe-4df3-854e-0d404a3a5f9a
[176] Microchips In Our Brains - Big Tech's A.I. Agenda
https://www.youtube.com/watch?v=hpcam2IQ1h8
Elon Musk's Neuralink brain chip demo explained
https://www.youtube.com/watch?v=KsX-7hS94Yo

willing to follow orders and subject their own populations to theft, atrocities, and even murder. Thus, the only way to confront such evil (actions from degraded personalities, rapacious greedy and or sociopathic personalities) is to oppose accepting such designs for the reshaping of society into essentially a global slave plantation, by opposing existing unethical social institutions and creating alternative social institutions based on human and environmental ethics. By rejecting the politics of anger, division, and hatred in favor of ethics and cooperation, by rejecting hierarchical technocratic digitized social prisons (facebook, twitter, youtube, cable news, corporate newspapers, and other propagandistic, censored social media), in favor of society based on ethics and truly sustainable relationships with humans, animals, and nature, the power, influence, and capacity to rule of the power elites is eroded. Of course, they will seek to ostracize, demonize, outlaw, etc., the dissenters, but what is the alternative, to be chattel slaves on the plantation of the neo-feudal slave plantation, without even freedom of thought? Here the importance of setting up communities with land and means of subsistence and joining with those who have the same goal of freedom of body, mind, and soul is important in order to avoid falling prey to the devolution of society and control by degraded personalities and their minions.

In this context, the power elites of today are the same kinds of personalities who attempted world domination throughout history such as Alexander, Attila, Napoleon, the Roman empire, the British empire, and the USA empire, etc. The present-day empire has seized on the opportunity, owing to advances in technology, to exert digital control worldwide. But the world is a large area and there are bound to be areas of resistance and alternative flourishing opportunities. Additionally, the global power elite plan has not been deployed without error and has not been able to be imposed universally, offering a situation where there are people who have had different experiences from what the power elite plan hoped. Many people have recognized the duplicity, the error, and the outright frauds being perpetrated by the supposed health agencies, the politicians and the media. Therefore, the designs of the global power elite are not infallible and not unopposed.

These areas of crisis can also be starting points for a strategy for those who want to seek to partner with peoples of like mind in order to provide better community, independent currency, natural living without digital bodily contaminations including 5G and Wi-Fi, promote ethical self-governance and an environment of positive spiritual evolution, regardless of what the future challenges may hold and regardless of the possible outcomes;-this is the right path.

FROM LOCKDOWNS TO VACCINE PASSPORTS TO COERCED VACCINATIONS.

Vaccine Passports Used To Create A Lesser Class of Citizens?[177]
•Apr 27, 2021

A doctor openly, on mainstream media, urges the president to use lockdowns to coerce the population into accepting vaccination. If lockdowns, as we now know, have no scientific evidence to support them but they are implemented anyway, what could be a purpose for their continued implementation by government officials? In the example above there is one possible answer to that question. Upon taking office the new president Biden stated he did not want to go the route of vaccine passports. Vaccine passports are the use of electronic records tracking those who have allowed themselves to be vaccinated to be allowed to participate fully in society and those not vaccinated being relegated to second class citizenship and loss of capacity to participate in previously freely available activities and benefits of society. However, why are certain personalities, including from the health sector, being allowed to go, unchallenged, on the mainstream media to float ideas such as that vaccine passports should be used as a "carrot" (meaning instrument of coercion) to get people to vaccinate so they can get their freedoms? And that the window is closing for the president to tie these two items, *passport and freedom*, together because states are reopening and people are going to experience their freedom and will not be able to be incentivized (coerced) to get the passports? So, in the TV cable program described above, there is also the admission that people can experience their freedoms without the passports; meaning that they do not need the passports to live normal lives but the opportunity to impose the unnecessary and ulterior motivated passports is closing, as people are moving, in varied locations and states around the country, to resume their lives, which proves people can live their lives without lockdowns and without vaccine passports. Furthermore, how is the

---

[177] https://www.youtube.com/watch?v=XUTM7c-Cz5o

ridiculous proposition by this doctor, that vaccinated people can gain their freedoms, supposed to be implemented anyway if even up to now people are being told, by the CDC and the president that they must still wear masks and social distance even after being vaccinated? Which freedoms is she referring to? Here we have an example of seemingly irrational, ridiculous statements and policy proposals that many people will latch on to and rush to get vaccinated only to find the so-called "carrot" was an illusion leading to no freedoms and more disease and more avenues of control, disempowerment, and impoverishments.

Over 1 Billion Worldwide Unwilling to Take COVID-19 Vaccine[178]

by Julie Ray May 3, 2021

This outing, by the doctor on a mainstream cable news show, is also a display of the political tactic of sending lower-ranked operatives to float certain ideas, in the public square, to see the mood of the electorate. It also serves the purpose of shaping the public mind. If not detected and confronted, such efforts can have a conditioning effect that adds up to manufacturing consent, in the public's mind, to the policies desired, even those that are against the interests of the public but for those of the power elites and their corporations. So, the higher officials did not say the words in the beginning so they do not have to confront opposition openly and foment mistrust or lose public support but if the ideas take hold then they can come out and support and implement them. This tactic is used especially with unpopular ideas or ideas that supposedly are for the public good that are in reality supporting industry and corporations.

Considering the brazen, and open exposition of the warped medical and power elite mindset of disregard for human individual sovereign rights and the perspective that arrogates to itself the right to dominate and coerce at will, the aforesaid is predicated on the idea that a person's human freedoms are dependent on an authority giving a passport and are not innate human freedoms without any passport at all.

Thus, lockdowns have an important purpose in support of vaccination efforts by governments. If the lockdowns can be maintained long enough or indefinitely, then people will be made sufficiently anxious (anxiety

---

[178] https://news.gallup.com/poll/348719/billion-unwilling-covid-vaccine.aspx

<u>DIGITAL PRISON CONSTRUCT</u> = Control of media + Control of the health industry + Control of the land and food industry +Control of Digital currency + tagging, tracing, monitoring through vaccines, smart devices with 5G and satellite surveillance

disorder) enough to accept being coerced into vaccinating if the reward is to be able to travel and have some semblance of "normalcy". Then, if vaccinations are successfully applied to the population it would be necessary to keep track of such vaccinated persons to know they are vaccinated versus those who are not. That would mean formalized tracking and surveillance, a "vaccine passport". Vaccine passports are a form of tracking and restriction on one hand, and coercion to force people to receive the experimental chemotherapies referred to as vaccines, along with social control. Therefore, lockdowns serve, among other things, the purpose of forcing people to accept vaccine regimes, to accept restriction of movements (no longer free), ease of police control, ease of future experimentation, and the acceptance of unknown chemical therapies that amount to human experiments with the possibility of early death and intentional forced population reduction.[179] Thus, vaccine passports are not gateways to freedom but rather to digital prison.

---

[179] https://articles.mercola.com/sites/articles/archive/2021/05/15/planet-lockdown.aspx?ui=152220df1deda081f73727bc10a8407027b248ba493a7ce71f4a1e73a6c1d882&sd=20200829&cid_source=dnl&cid_medium=email&cid_content=art1HL&cid=20210515&mid=DM885052&rid=1158339911

'Freedom' pass | France wants to be first EU state to bring in Covid passports
•Apr 22, 2021[180]

UK wants to introduce vaccine passports by mid-May
•Apr 22, 2021

Prime Minister Boris Johnson has indicated he wants them to be ready by May 17th.[181]

The imposition of lockdowns has produced a situation whereby the population has been dispossessed and impoverished, facilitating a financial coup of the corporations and the rich to acquire and control business and real estate wealth assets and at the same time thwarting the capacity for populist political movements.

The elements have been put in place over decades but in the year 2020 they were activated, in an apparent coordinated manner, so as to have an activated formula for the imposition of a "digital prison" by the global power elites.

A Strategy of ignorant protests or strategic civil disobedience

The coronavirus "crisis" that has been affecting countries the world over has been revealed as a pseudo-pandemic and a premeditated false-flag event to be used to panic the world population and facilitate overturning individual national autonomy and sovereignty and facilitating worldwide fascist control by forcing a health crisis and destroying the previous economic model. Now, in the wake of the forced pandemic, forced fear and destitution due to unlawful and unscientific lockdowns that close businesses, the central banking system

---

[180] https://on.rt.com/b6hp
[181] https://www.euronews.com/2021/04/22/u...

and bought off politicians are poised to take over the bankrupt populations while ~~printing,~~ rather, counterfeiting currency, to buy bankrupted businesses and resources for the corporate elite.

The protests and suffering of the population under rapacious capitalism and neoliberal corporate socio-political economics under the democratic party rule and the corporate neoconservative corruptions of the republican party rule have both led to the impoverishment and suffering of the population domestically and have, as well, forced wars and coup d'etats around the world. Having achieved control of the media in a digital age, the ruling class, through government agencies and tech companies, has imposed propaganda on the population leading to mistrust by the population which is so psychologically and physically debilitated and diseased, so fearful and dumbed down as to go along with the dictates of the government and corporate elites even after finding their directives to be based on lies. The decades of impoverishment and exploitation under corporate government (fascism-union of corporations and the democrat and republican parties) and no relief or justice from the government, have also fostered, stoked, and exacerbated existing, anger, anxiety, fears, and disbelief of real conspiracies between corporations and government officials, while stoking belief in unproven conspiracy theories such as "Qanon". Adding to those factors are the real racial tensions due to past and present injustices, and ignorance in the population which lead to greater conflict between subgroups of the population and between the population and the government.

The protests at the US Capitol on Jan 6th, which were carried out at the insistence of Donald Trump and were attended by many disgruntled people including disenfranchised workers and people who are tired of lies and corruption in politics and the media. It was as well attended by nativists, bigots, and racists as well as smaller groups who meant to use the opportunity to foment discord and violence (possible operatives from the CIA and FBI). The protest was apparently also attended by members of the police that were in league with or sympathetic to the protest and assisted it. A few days after the incident the democrat politicians and later joined by the cable media and social media started an echo chamber of labeling all the participants (perhaps up to 1000 US citizens) as "domestic" terrorists. In the following weeks, they started repeating the idea that those people, some of which voted for Donald Trump out of spite for the democratic and corporate elite corruptions and others who believed in his white supremacist and misogynist rhetoric should be treated like terrorists who need to be "deprogrammed" or even "droned"[182]. Also, calls (floating a policy to shape the public mind and facilitate legislation) started to go out for a new "patriot act" stile escalation of surveillance and censorship that already had begun with censorship actions imposed by tech companies on social media. It is now clear that the social media tech companies are in league with the neoliberal politicians, controlling the democratic party, in promoting propaganda and censoring dissenting views in the media and anywhere in society, which will be assisted by propagandized members of the population itself. So the protest is being used as an opportunity, not to consider or review why there is growing racism, sexism, hatred, fear, mistrust, and aggression towards others, politicians, between ethnic groups, etc.; rather, the opportunity is being seized to expand government control, stoke more fear for manipulation and control and expand the police state to the level of a mass surveillance police state which could be followed by expanded mass incarceration without any due process but by decree. This kind of development signals the suspension/rescinding of human inalienable rights and only sustains the rights and privilages of the elites and the relatively privileged technocratic positions of those who assist them or do not openly disagree with them. Such a state of society is called totalitarianism and its economic system may be characterized as neo-feudalism. Thus, while people within a society might be concerned with social issues such as racism, sexism, abortion, etc. the power elite do not care about such issues personally; rather, those issues, which are endemic in spiritually and socially degraded societies, are used to stoke division, and discontent so as to be a distraction from the agenda of totalitarian dispossession of rights and wealth that the power elite are perpetrating on the population as a whole. The dispossession of rights (suspension or cancellation of the rule of law) and wealth inequality are hallmarks of totalitarianism and neo-feudalism. **A Strategy of ignorant protests or *misdirected or aimless* civil disobedience** that does not take into account the higher objectives and goal of the power elite and which does not confront the power elites, both on judicial and legislative grounds, will be ineffective and will actually work to the advantage of the power elites.

---

[182] https://www.youtube.com/watch?v=aU5hw9H7htc

Protests and Socio-political-economic Change

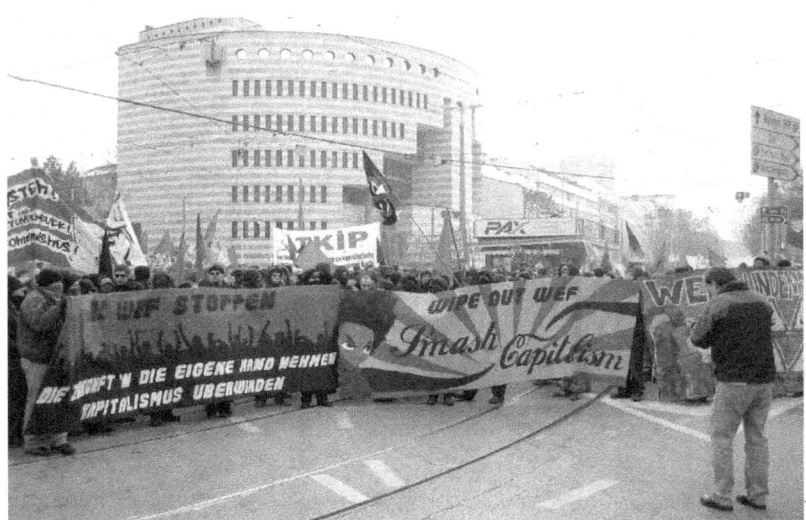

Protest march against the World Economic Forum in Basel, 2006. Photo by Hanno Böck - Selbst fotografiert in Basel

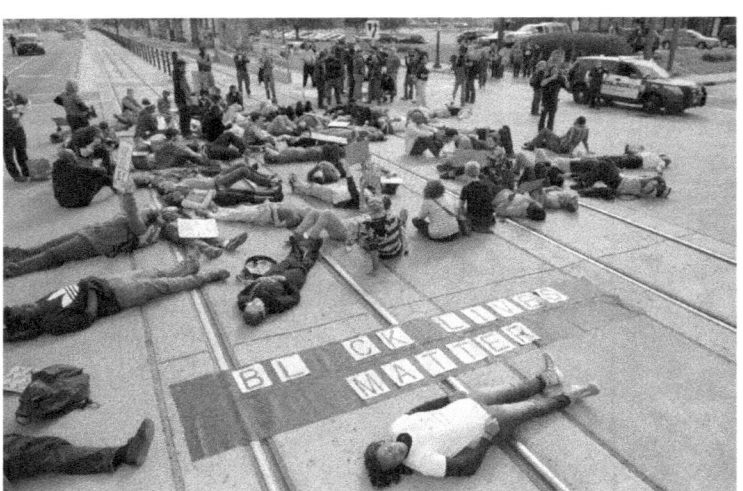

A Black Lives Matter die-in over rail tracks, protesting alleged police brutality in Saint Paul, Minnesota (September 20, 2015)

> St. Paul, Minnesota September 20, 2015, Around 100 protesters blocked the light rail line in St. Paul to protest the treatment of Marcus Abrams by St. Paul police. Abrams, who is 17 and has Autism, was violently arrested by Metro Transit Police on August 31, 2015. During his arrest,

he suffered a split lip and multiple seizures. The letter A on their sign fell off on the march. On the march back, a small cheer went up when someone found it, and the march paused while it was re-attached. 2015-09-20 This is licensed under a Creative Commons Attribution License. Photo by Fibonacci Blue

The BLM Effect: Study Shows Police Killings Dropped as Much as 20 Percent In Cities After Black Lives Matter Protests[183]
March 8, 2021

US Capitol Protest on Jan 6, 2021

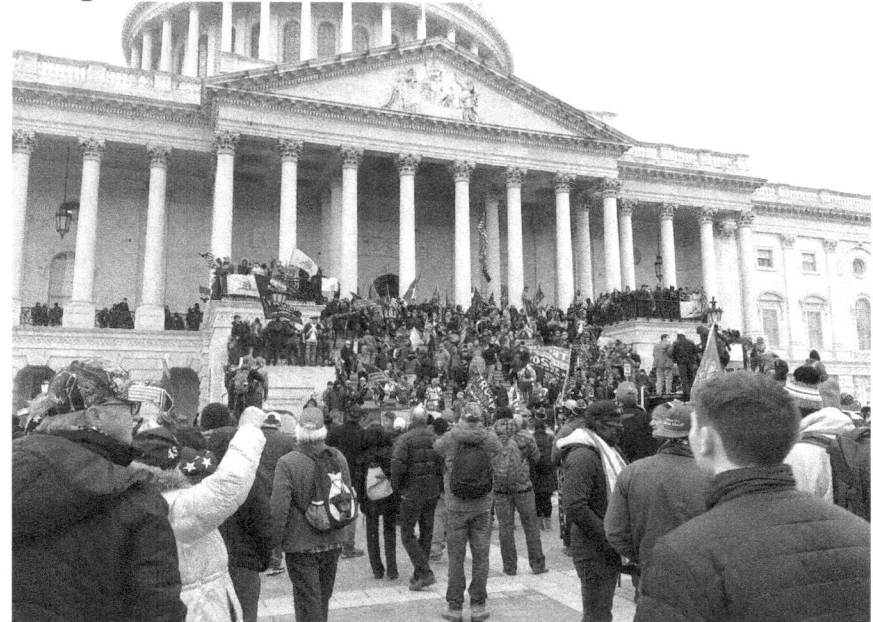

Image of a crowd of Trump supporters marching on the US Capitol on 6 January 2021, ultimately leading to the building being breached and several deaths.[184]

The protests that occurred at the US Capitol on Jan 6, 2021, are an example of the level of discontent, angst, and disgust with the political system and power elite paradigm under which all are forced

---

[183] HTTPS://ATLANTABLACKSTAR.COM/2021/03/08/THE-BLM-EFFECT-STUDY-SHOWS-POLICE-KILLINGS-DROPPED-AS-MUCH-AS-20-PERCENT-IN-CITIES-AFTER-BLACK-LIVES-MATTER-PROTESTS/
[184] https://en.wikipedia.org/wiki/2021_storming_of_the_United_States_Capitol#/media/File:DC_Capitol_Storming_IMG_7986.jpg

to live. Journalist Joe Lauria had some important insights (excerpts below) about how the power elite mainstream media tried to portray the incident and how people in congress also tried to characterize the event so as to invalidate and dismiss its significance so as to continue corrupt business as usual, while at the same time drumming u an excuse for having a reason to put down the protests and increase police state powers to do violence and more surveillance on the people as well as any of like mind including those who voted for Donald Trump.

Capitol Incident a Dress Rehearsal
January 8, 2021 [185]

The problem of protests by the ignorant and fearful is that they fall into the hands of those in control of the levers of power justifying their use of deadly force to put down the protests. Such protests occur because, in part, people feel there is no other option. That is the case because ordinary citizens are not able to effect change through traditional political mechanisms, as those have been bought off by the power elite. Ordinary citizens, being compromised by ignorance, pleasure-seeking, belief and trust in the corrupt leaders, belief and trust in the corrupt capitalist-power elite system and being weakened by living life without ethical conscience, they cannot otherwise do other tactical moves that would be substantive and helpful towards the building and sustaining of a society based on ethics and caring for all. Some of those tactics might include: stopping supporting the power elites and the corporations and paying taxes to corrupt government officials, practicing civil disobedience in order to obstruct the operations of the power elites and the fascist collusion with government technocrats.

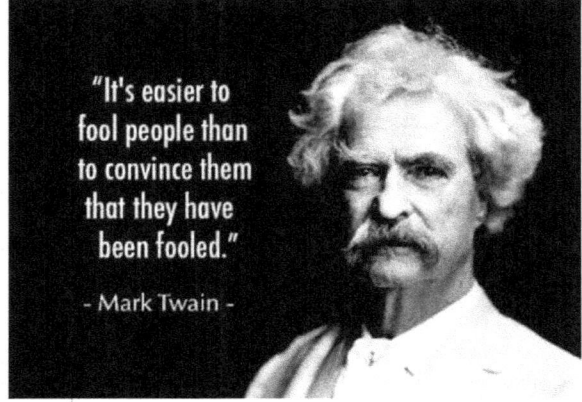

[185] https://consortiumnews.com/2021/01/08/capitol-incident-a-dress-rehearsal/

Since people are too weak to move out of their comfort zones in order to collectively oppose injustices, by continually voting for the lesser of two evils, the evils get progressively worse and only those whose angst can barely be contained take to the streets flailing irrationally, thereby accomplishing little for themselves but plenty for the power structure and their propaganda machine that characterizes the protests as unpatriotic rebellious attempts. While protests are necessary to confront evil, those should be a strategic part of an overall strategy including seeking self-reliance and stopping supporting the power elite and government injustices and instead of reforming and taking control of the government through civil disobedience and then establishing an order based on ethics and the application of the unbiased laws to the corporations and power elites along with everyone else. These strategies should be implemented while taking care not to fall into the hands of the power structure that is eager for people to do acts of desperation so as to use that as an excuse to call them radicals and then proceed, with that justification, to discredit their efforts and use the pain, caused by the leaders, to label the sufferers as "unpatriotic and or agents of chaos or violence" and then impose more draconian force to suppress their outcries and protests. This was an important lesson learned from the OCCUPY WALLSTREET PROTEST MOVEMENT. Protests should be part of a SOCIO-POLITICAL strategy leading to real political power, that can counteract the designs of the power elites, and not goals in and of themselves. Protests, as part of an overall strategy, can serve to let all members of the society know about an issue so that those of like mind may join the cause. However, they cannot accomplish the full goal of reform or revolution on their own. If not used wisely they can become sources of exacerbation of the problems of the society, in terms of stress and strife and then also they can play into the hands of the power elite corrupted paradigm of demonization by the corporate-owned mainstream and social media. That is then followed by police action that puts the protests down, often with the approval of the public that the protests were intended to help. Then they are followed by marginalization and political impotence.

The issue, about the plight of the masses, the ill-thought-out protesting, the possible derailment due to agent provocateurs, and the possibility of provoking an outsized negative reaction from the power elite power structure controlling the power centers of society was outlined by investigative journalist Allan Nairn[186]:

---

[186] "AMERICANS ARE NOW GETTING A MILD TASTE OF THEIR OWN MEDICINE" OF DISRUPTING DEMOCRACY ELSEWHERE

"Americans Are Now Getting a Mild Taste of Their Own Medicine" of Disrupting Democracy Elsewhere

Story January 07, 2021 [187]

Dr. Joseph Mercola outlines the result of the seemingly irrational but well developed and intentionally tyrannical policies imposed on the world human population.

Public Health Officials Are Destroying Humanity

Story at-a-glance [188]

---

[187] https://www.democracynow.org/2021/1/7/us_foreign_election_interference_allan_nairn
[188] https://articles.mercola.com/sites/articles/archive/2021/02/11/lockdown.aspx?ui=152220df1deda081f73727bc10a8407027b248ba493a7ce71f4a1e73a6c1d882&sd=20200829&cid_source=dnl&cid_medium=email&cid_content=art1HL&cid=20210211&mid=DM801843&rid=1081645302

The Dire Prospects for the Future of Human Society and the Challenges Ahead for Successful Spiritual Life and Working Towards a Better World

What began as secret universal wiretapping under the Clinton and Bush presidencies, after the attacks of 9/11/01, developed further with the Patriot Act under president Obama leading to secret illegal information sharing among US government agencies including FBI, NSA, CIA, and local police. Surveillance increased through smartphones and smart devices, social media interactions profiling and now (2021) there are plans to increase surveillance to facial recognition and other biometrics. Additionally, "vaccine" company producers have talked about including particles in vaccines to track people. Thus, the western countries and north-America in particular (USA and Canada), have become the most heavily surveilled populations in history, except perhaps considering China.

It is therefore apparent that a new phase of the USA police state that was previously considered to be "soft" has moved into a "new phase" that includes hard and open censorship, hard as well as open propaganda and censorship, which will continue to escalate to further polarization, militarization, divisions and social conflict which may escalate to open conflict, martial law, and disintegration of society. This is due to the fact that the neoliberal politicians and their followers, the democratic party, are poised to demonize those who voted against them and they seem undaunted in the program of impoverishment, exploitation, and rapacious capitalism for the power elite that are controlling them from the commanding heights of the economy, the central banks, and through organizations such as WHO, World Bank, IMF, and World Economic Forum / Davos, etc. under the guise of a benevolent "Great Reset".

TWO POWER ELITE SPONSORED GREAT RESETS FACING THE WORLD POPULATIONS

There are two "resets" being discussed. One is the reset of the dying US Dollar to a digital currency for continued and expanding economic exploitation of the economy for banking interests and the banking power elites; this is the financial and monetary great reset. The second "great reset" is being touted by the World Economic Forum, a group of power elites that want to reset human culture itself supposedly for the betterment of humanity, tackling the problems of climate change and inequality, for example. This is the social and political "great reset". However, their own statements and publications, attest to their ulterior motives which are directed at the benefit of the power elite by wresting control over and impoverishing world populations, industry, culture, and nature itself as a whole.

This being the case, it is recommended that the reader should see the references listed, in this document, examining the information with an open mind and with a view of facing the challenges of life with honesty, and then take appropriate actions to protect family and wealth, support ethics and righteousness in society when possible, and be sure to follow the protocols of physical health and spiritual life. This means striving to live by ethics, critical thinking and seeking to know information outside of mainstream censorship outlets, the responsibility to support resistance to injustices such as lockdowns supposedly imposed to help reduce the coronavirus disease but which science proves have no positive effect and promote more injuries and deaths as well as a pandemics of fear[189]. (Examples of such protests include: as in –Mexico,[190] Italy,[191] Denmark[192]). Other actions have been mentioned earlier, that reduce dependency on the power elite institutions,

---

[189] https://duckduckgo.com/?t=ffab&q=standford+lockdowns&ia=web
https://www.lifesitenews.com/news/stanford-study-lockdowns-have-no-significant-effect-in-reducing-covid-19-may-even-spread-it
[190] https://duckduckgo.com/?q=Mexico+protest+lockdown&t=ffab&ia=web
https://fronterasdesk.org/content/1650800/armed-pans-and-spoons-restaurants-mexico-city-protest-against-lockdown
[191] https://off-guardian.org/2021/01/15/i-am-open-50000-italian-restaurant-owners-plan-to-ignore-lockdown/
[192] https://duckduckgo.com/?q=denmark+protest+cancel+vaccine&t=ffab&ia=web
https://duckduckgo.com/?q=denmark+protest+cancel+vaccine&t=ffab&ia=web

including the purchase of gold and silver, preparing for life and survival in social breakdown conditions, etc.

MEDICAL MARTIAL LAW AND MEDICAL EMERGENCIES AS TOOLS TO ALLOW THE POWER ELITE TO USHER IN TOTALITARIANISM.

MEDICAL MARTIAL LAW 2020[193]

During the anthrax scare of 2001 and the emergence of the previous SARS Covid pandemic scare of the early 2000s, governments around the world, especially in North America and Europe, have been implementing incremental acts and laws that have added up to effective "Medical Martial Law." "Medical tyranny" or "Medical Martial Law" is the idea of having laws and regulations that supersede the laws enacted by popular elections and due processes that citizens are involved with. Medical Martial Laws are acts enacted by bureaucrats and unelected health officials using a supposed public health crisis to suspend civil liberties and have the power to impose regulations that would be ordinary and normal in a totalitarian state but not in a truly free or democratic society where people determine the laws they will govern themselves by. Medical Martial Law accomplishes the goal of authoritarian personalities and or groups (the power elite) for totalitarian control of a population without the objections, protests and dissent from the population, that would occur if there were an overt Coup d'état or a decree of Martial Law by politicians or a military officer.

---

[193] https://www.corbettreport.com/medical-martial-law-2020/

> https://swprs.org/the-trouble-with-pcr-tests/
>
> Already in mid-March, SPR explained that the highly sensitive PCR tests are prone to producing false-positive results and their individual predictive value may easily drop below 50%.
>
>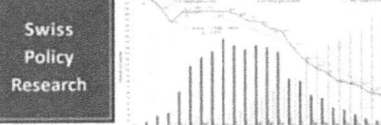
>
> But if there is an ongoing infection wave, or if there has been a recent infection wave, or if labs test only for one gene sequence or struggle with contamination, things get more complicated.
>
> A PCR test is amplifying samples through repetitive cycles. The lower the virus concentration in the sample, the more cycles are needed to achieve a positive result. Many US labs work with 35 to 45 cycles, while many European labs work with 30 to 40 cycles.
>
> The research group of French professor Didier Raoult has recently shown that at a cycle threshold (ct) of 25, about 70% of samples remained positive in cell culture (i.e. were infectious); at a ct of 30, 20% of samples remained positive; at a ct of 35, 3% of samples remained positive; and at a ct above 35, no sample remained positive (infectious) in cell culture (see diagram).
>
> This means that if a person gets a "positive" PCR test result at a cycle threshold of 35 or higher (as applied in most US labs and many European labs), the chance that the person is infectious is less than 3%. The chance that the person received a "false positive" result is 97% or higher.

The continued use of known fraudulent and discredited PCR,[194] test (for determination of coronavirus infection) as an excuse to call an official "pandemic" and scare populations about a supposed "health crisis", and statements by the supposed health authorities, like Dr. Fauci, supported by government officials like president Biden, continuing to support the existence of a pandemic on that basis is a fraud on the population. Further, after the coronavirus disease proved to be no worse than the FLU and the general population has at least 99.5% chance of not being affected (affects only .5% -at most-of the population)-which means there was and is no pandemic and therefore no need for emergency measures but still there is a continued push for the administration of a so-called vaccines; and those vaccines, even after being taken, offer no assurance of not contracting, passing on, or dying from the supposed coronavirus pandemic disease points to ulterior motivations.

---

[194] https://www.drbvip.com/
https://youtu.be/Q9GccuvNs9U

Covid-19 Vaccine	age group	Survival Rate without a comorbid condition
• Does NOT Provide Immunity		
• Does NOT Eliminate the Virus		
• Does NOT Prevent Death		
• Does NOT Prevent infection	under 1	99.993%
• Does NOT Prevent Transmission	1 yr-4yr	99.988%
• Does NOT Eliminate Mask wearing	5yr-14yr	99.967%
• Does NOT Eliminate Anti-social distancing	15yr-24yrs	99.93%
• Does NOT Eliminate Travel Bans	25 yrs-34yrs	99.82%
• Does NOT Eliminate Business Closures	35yrs-44yrs	99.68%
• Does NOT Eliminate Lockdowns	45 yrs-54yrs	99.54%
	55yrs-64yrs	99.52%
Covid-19 vaccine	65yrs-74yrs	99.5%
• Is NOT FDA Approved	75yrs-84yrs	99.5%
• Has NO Liability	85yrs and over	99.5%
• No Long Term Studies		
• No Studies on Patients with Comorbid Conditions		

[195]

Also, the contradiction that even after taking the experimental vaccines people still would need to wear masks, socially distance and continue lockdowns points to futile, empty acts by people in response to the disease but are unwitting acts in support of a "fear appeal" strategy being perpetrated on the population. Added to all of that is the scare over the supposed emergence of "new" supposedly more dangerous coronavirus "variants" (that were later discovered to be already in the population months earlier and were no more dangerous) –all this now signals that the "authorities" intend to continue imposing the wearing of masks, socially distancing and continue lockdowns indefinitely along with contact tracing, to monitor the population. This state of affairs, a pandemic scare environment with the excuse of being able to tell people not to gather in large groups, effectively shuts down the kinds of assembly, protest, and dissent, which are necessary avenues to discuss, evaluate and formulate responses to political situations such as oppression, exploitation and government illegality while granting social dominance to the power elite and the unelected bureaucrats indefinitely; that is because the excuse of a supposed health crisis could potentially be indefinite since viruses are part of the worldwide human environment and will therefore always be around in some form or another. Another issue is that since the covid 19 virus was apparently created or developed in a lab in Wuhan China with the help of experiments conducted at Ft. Dietrich and the University of North Carolina and funded by the head of the U.S. National Institute of Allergy and

---

[195] drbvip.com/

Infectious Diseases (Anthony Fauci, the same person charged with responding to the supposed virus), the possible unintentional release or intentional weaponizing[196] and release of viruses and their variants that can exist is only limited to the capacity for their unknown production. China and the USA have now both been found to be doing secret experimentation to weaponize infectious agents. The concern over the US government agencies experimenting with and releasing pathogens is not unprecedented since the US government has been found to be spreading infections agents to the unknowing public, for purposes of germ warfare testing.[197]

Chinese document discussing weaponizing coronaviruses provides 'chilling' information
•May 9, 2021

==============

Dr. Fauci Backed Controversial Wuhan Lab with U.S. Dollars for Risky Coronavirus Research[198]
By Fred Guterl On 4/28/20

---

[196] Sky News Australia- https://youtu.be/kuKPBur_TiI
[197] https://www.instagram.com/tv/COj8H7Qn4wV/?igshid=qyh1i1677acr
[198] https://www.newsweek.com/dr-fauci-backed-controversial-wuhan-lab-millions-us-dollars-risky-coronavirus-research-1500741

BREAKING: KENNEDY EXPOSES DR. FAUCI'S ROLE IN CREATING HIGHLY INFECTIOUS MUTANT STRAIN OF CORONAVIRUS

By Robert F. Kennedy Jr.

===========

Center for Food Safety Sues NIH Over Unlawfully Keeping Secret Federal Funding of Research Creating New More Virulent Pandemic Viruses

NIH Failed to Promptly Release Documents Concerning "Gain of Function/Gain of Threat" Research on Influenza, MERS, SARS, and COVID
May 04, 2021

THE FRAUD OF VACCINE EFFICACY

Dr. Ron Brown Discusses Outcome Reporting Bias in COVID-19 mRNA Clinical Trials Interview[199]

Dr. Ron Brown discusses the danger of outcome reporting bias and the misleading conclusions and violations of informed consent from outcome reporting bias in COVID-19 mRNA vaccine clinical trials.

Evidence emerged about how the world population was fooled into believing the pharmaceutical company chemical gene therapies called "vaccines" are efficacious against the disease referred to as "coronavirus" or "covid 19". Dr. Fauci, FDA, government officials, medical workers, and the media have been misleading the public about the disease referred to as "coronavirus" or "covid 19" being "more lethal" than the annual FLU, about the infection fatality rate, and the case fatality rate, and the vaccine efficacy. Initially, before deploying the vaccines to the public the data from the tests that was released from the pharmaceutical companies, and was publicized in the mainstream media, was that the covid

---

[199] https://youtu.be/Jkwn5I8tLmE

19 vaccine efficacy rates were 90% or 95%, etc. Those numbers made headlines and was repeated by politicians, supposed health officials, and the media followed by general ignorant health workers including clinicians, nurses, etc. The figures used to arrive at those high success rates were not released before the deployment started.

After the numbers used to arrive at those high calculations were released, Dr. Ron Brown arrived at efficacy rates that are nowhere near 90%. The true efficacy rates are a dismal failure. Yet, the fraudulent figures that were initially given to the media, are still repeated by the supposed health agencies, the politicians, and the media. Therefore, the chemical gene therapies touted as "vaccines" are a major fraud being perpetrated on the world population. <u>The actual absolute efficacy rates of the so-called "vaccines" for coronavirus are: 0.7% for the Pfizer chemical gene therapy injection touted as "vaccine" and 1.1% for the Moderna chemical gene therapy injection touted as "vaccine"</u>.[200] These misrepresentations by the WHO, CDC, NIH, the president, the media, and the pharmaceutical companies fostered fear in the public, diminution of the public's capacity to think rationally about the risks of the disease, the risk vs. benefit of so-called ineffective and apparently dangerous vaccines, and apparently intentionally led to fear-based faith in a supposed "effective", "vaccine" cure and or preventative for the disease referred to as "coronavirus" or "covid 19". Another fraud pointed out by Dr. Ron Brown is fact that the health officials knew about the fact that lockdowns did not help china and that there would be deaths by collateral damage caused by the fear and lockdowns. At the very least these revelations mean that the health officials are untrustworthy; Moreover, it also means they perpetrated the deceptions to lead people away from alternative supplements and drugs and to the lucrative supposed "vaccines". Additionally, they are likely criminally responsible for the collateral deaths caused by their misrepresentations of the disease, lockdowns, and deaths from the so-called vaccines themselves.

As of April and continuing into May 2021, the vaccine Adverse Reaction data has demonstrated unequivocal indications that the chemical gene therapies referred to as "vaccines" are ***not*** safe or effective.[201] Other emerging pieces of evidence are now also showing "breakthrough cases", which means people are contracting covid 19 disease after being

---

[200] ibid
[201] Dr. Jessica Rose "A report on the U.S. Adverse Events Reporting System (VAERS) of the COVID-19 Messenger RNA (mRNA) biologicals" https://youtu.be/CfeiZzXcjNw

"vaccinated."[202] Additionally, more evidence is suggesting that the chemical gene therapies referred to as "vaccines" cause prion disease. Further evidence suggests that the new "vaccines" have potential dangers for the non-vaccinated, due to shedding,[203] and maybe causing reproductive organ damage and miscarriages[204] and may also cause infertility in men and women.[205] Also, due to shedding, it is possible that the chemical gene therapies called "vaccines" could partially transfer from the injected persons to those who did not receive the pseudo-vaccines and if that were to occur those people's reproductive capacity could be affected, along with the host of other vaccine adverse reactions that could occur especially if they have co-morbid conditions. This last point would raise the suspicion that the vaccine was designed to operate in this way, thereby purposefully affecting the general population, among other reasons, to cause infertility and promote a depopulation agenda. The implications of the latter point could have far-reaching social, legal, and political ramifications and that should trigger the convening of a new Nuremberg Tribunal[206] for the crimes of:

1- doing the GAIN OF FUNCTION experiments to make a deadly virus –essentially a biological weapon that escaped a lab by accident or by design,
2-interfering by dictating which treatments doctors should use and which not,
3-telling the population that there is no treatment (when there are proven safe and effective treatments) and to wait at home for vaccines, and in the meantime allowing 10s of thousands to die,
4- locking down society with no scientific proof and destroying the economy and peoples economic lives,
5-convincing people through propaganda that the experimental vaccines are safe and effective,
6-censoring debate and information disproving the claims of safety and effectiveness of the experimental vaccines,
7-administering experimental vaccines without informed consent.

---

[202] Dr. John Bergman www.drbvip.com
[203] Dr. John Bergman www.drbvip.com
Dr. Christiane Northrup | New Details on C-19 Injections
https://brandnewtube.com/v/TdDZQw
[204] https://humansarefree.com/2021/03/miscarriages-increase-by-366-due-to-covid-vaccines.html
[205] Dr. Christiane Northrup | New Details on C-19 Injections
 https://brandnewtube.com/v/TdDZQw
[206] Nuremberg Tribunal https://nuremberg.law.harvard.edu/

These violations can be considered crimes against humanity. Without this kind of response, there will be impunity that will allow the continuation of the crimes that could lead to the deaths of large numbers of people (billions).

> "Everything your government and their advisors have said about the pandemic is untrue."
> —Dr. Michael Yeadon[207]

The Nuremberg Code (1947)

Permissible Medical Experiments

The great weight of the evidence before us to effect that certain types of medical experiments on human beings, when kept within reasonably well-defined bounds, conform to the ethics of the medical profession generally. The protagonists of the practice of human experimentation justify their views on the basis that such experiments yield results for the good of society that are unprocurable by other methods or means of study. All agree, however, that certain basic principles must be observed in order to satisfy moral, ethical and legal concepts:

1. The voluntary consent of the human subject is absolutely essential. This means that the person involved should have legal capacity to give consent; should be so situated as to be able to exercise free power of choice, without the intervention of any element of force, fraud, deceit, duress, overreaching, or other ulterior form of constraint or coercion; and should have sufficient knowledge and comprehension of the elements of the subject matter involved as to enable him to make an understanding and enlightened decision. This latter element requires that before the acceptance of an affirmative decision by the experimental subject there should be made known to him the nature, duration, and purpose of the experiment; the method and means by which it is to be conducted; all inconveniences and hazards reasonably to be expected; and the effects upon his health or person which may possibly come from his participation in the experiment.

The duty and responsibility for ascertaining the quality of the consent rests upon each individual who initiates, directs, or engages in the experiment. It is

---

[207] https://youtu.be/Ay12R0e_7WM

a personal duty and responsibility which may not be delegated to another with impunity.

2. The experiment should be such as to yield fruitful results for the good of society, unprocurable by other methods or means of study, and not random and unnecessary in nature.

3. The experiment should be so designed and based on the results of animal experimentation and a knowledge of the natural history of the disease or other problem under study that the anticipated results justify the performance of the experiment.

4. The experiment should be so conducted as to avoid all unnecessary physical and mental suffering and injury.

5. No experiment should be conducted where there is an a priori reason to believe that death or disabling injury will occur; except, perhaps, in those experiments where the experimental physicians also serve as subjects.

6. The degree of risk to be taken should never exceed that determined by the humanitarian importance of the problem to be solved by the experiment.

7. Proper preparations should be made and adequate facilities provided to protect the experimental subject against even remote possibilities of injury, disability or death.

8. The experiment should be conducted only by scientifically qualified persons. The highest degree of skill and care should be required through all stages of the experiment of those who conduct or engage in the experiment.

9. During the course of the experiment the human subject should be at liberty to bring the experiment to an end if he has reached the physical or mental state where continuation of the experiment seems to him to be impossible.

10. During the course of the experiment the scientist in charge must be prepared to terminate the experiment at any stage, if he has probable cause to believe, in the exercise of the good faith, superior skill and careful judgment required of him, that a continuation of the experiment is likely to result in injury, disability, or death to the experimental subject.

For more information see Nuremberg Doctor's Trial, *BMJ* 1996;313(7070):1445-75.

That capacity, of gain of function research scientists around the world, to release more viruses, whenever desired could fuel the excuse for the supposed need of indefinite time of mask-wearing, social distancing, etc. and indefinite numbers of "vaccines" and indefinite time of Medical Martial Law; that is, unless the population wises up to the fraudulent agenda and rises in opposition to the sociopathic attempts to enslave the world population in a global totalitarian digital surveillance police state, which is the desired "new normal" by the power elites, that otherwise will be accepted, if not demanded by the ignorant, angst afflicted population.[208] Due to the imposition of fear, propaganda, censorship, and intentional or unintentional conflicting public health and government directives, over time, people become so confused and anxious that their capacity for rational thought will be so damaged that they themselves will call for medical martial law to protect them and they will accept the controls and injustices willingly.

> In the foreword to the 1946 edition of his novel, **Brave New World**, Aldous Huxley anticipated the continued emergence, perhaps in novel forms, of statist totalitarianism:[209]

Aldous Huxley also described what he was seeing in his time, which has developed up to our time, an emergence of totalitarianism that is to be achieved by essentially throwing out the norms and ethics by which world culture was, if not following, was at least guided by in the past. The new paradigm is of corrupting, inverting those norms, and using those same norms to subvert their goals. Instead of past norms such as the ideal of equality, the ideal of equality would be professed but the policies would foster inequality. Here also, the norm of democracy and republican representative government is distorted so as to have the appearance of democracy and republican representative government while achieving instead an autocratic totalitarian outcome. So, while making the appearance, but not the substance, of ethics, humanitarianism, and goodwill, the real outcome, is economic disparity, social polarization, and rogue

---

[208] https://www.corbettreport.com/mml2020/
https://www.youtube.com/watch?v=Q9GccuvNs9U
https://youtu.be/EWNkJUDctdk
[209] https://www.sgtreport.com/2021/01/huxleys-warning-totalitarianism-in-the-21st-century/

government. Such a "turned around" version of totalitarianism was envisioned by the political philosopher Sheldon Wolin. [210]

> The political philosopher Sheldon Wolin coined the term inverted totalitarianism in 2003 to describe what he saw as the emerging form of government of the United States.
>
> The book Days of Destruction, Days of Revolt (2012) by Chris Hedges and Joe Sacco portrays inverted totalitarianism as a system where corporations have corrupted and subverted democracy and where economics bests politics.

Wolin's analysis in 2008 traced the development from the time of authors such as George Orwell and Aldus Huxley of a relentless move towards totalitarian rule. Wolin's assessment of the USA government as developing into inverted totalitarianism is the culmination of what the previous authors envisioned. The power of technology and the capacity to miseducate and confuse the masses through mass propaganda[211], and censorship, playing on the innate human fears and cognitive flaws such as hereditary tendency to defer to authority, normalcy bias, cognitive dissonance, and the immature need to belong to and be accepted by a social group, regardless of ethics. Those human flaws facilitate delusions, coercions, miseducations and manipulations, and the imposition of totalitarian policies in an unprecedented manner, not possible by would-be tyrants of the past, with the help of modern technology. Therefore, there should be no expectation that those who have arrived at the threshold of totalitarian power and control will ever want to give it up and have to stop imposing the policies of control and with them the fear-mongering that supports it. In this context, coronavirus could be seen as a perfect invisible enemy that, unlike the fictitious weapons of mass destruction that were the excuse for invading Iraq, by imposing propaganda and censorship in the USA about the evidence, etc., the coronavirus is, in a way, an "invisible" "enemy" that causes visible harm, and can be perpetual and whose deadliness can be revived and amplified or reduced at will like the danger color code used following the 911 attacks, as a barometer, whenever the need arises to raise the tensions and anxieties of a population to bend their will to the totalitarian designs. For example, a new supposedly more virulent "variant" can be released to re-scare populations into submission. Or, by using the fraudulent

---

[210] Wolin, Sheldon S. (2008). *Democracy Incorporated: Managed Democracy and the Specter of Inverted Totalitarianism*. Princeton: Princeton University Press. ISBN 0-691-13566-5.
[211] https://youtu.be/Pfo5gPG72KM

PCR test to scare people into believing that there are "new surges of infected cases" and then imposing new lockdowns and mask wearing and then relaxing those regulations and then reinstituting the regulations, the stress and fear levels of the population can be manipulated for the fascist goals. **NOTE:** Viruses normally do not become more virulent as they move through a population. They do normally mutate as they move through a population, varying 1-3% from the original and the variants have not been found to be more dangerous than the original. The existence of variants can be used to scare people but the scientific finding is that the variants are not sufficiently different from the original to be a cause for new concern though the health officials and media and politicians try to use the existence of variants as a means to scare people into accepting more loss of rights, control, and vaccines.[212] Thus, by finding new "variants" a supposedly temporary state of emergency could be restarted and maintained, at will, in perpetuity, justifying new lockdowns and scares with the excuse of the invisible, though in reality not lethal, enemy that they own the patents and tests for. Thus, it is incumbent upon all thoughtful persons, with the capacity of determining self-will, to act in a manner such that their security, body autonomy, and mental health would be best protected and served.

A Scientist Speaks out on the Issue of Covid 19 Variants

Prof. Luc Montagnier: "Variants come from vaccinations"[213]

---

[212] https://www.bitchute.com/video/q1SooK2qbRg4/
[213] https://planetes360.fr/pr-luc-montagnier-les-variants-viennent-des-vaccinations/

LOOKING AHEAD: 2021 AND BEYOND

The supposed medical protection agencies of the USA including the CDC, supposed health agencies, NIAID, NIH, CDC, etc. have been found to be laden with conflicts of interest, corruption, profit motive, and purposeful miseducation, and misleading the public for their own gain, which has been a development not of recent origins but over decades. The covid 19 scares have caused mass panic and hysteria throughout the world with the apparent goal of a mass, worldwide, set of injections with experimental and increasingly provable dangerous chemical gene therapy drugs. The covid 19 scare is apparently being used to usher in the 'new world order' envisioned by the power elites, of complete digital control through vaccine passports and possible mass depopulation[214] (genocide). Clearly, the apparent strategy is to maintain the covid 19 scare indefinitely and make the medical tyranny more into medical martial law. The medical martial law is therefore the vehicle for fearmongering, impoverishment through lockdowns, vaccine passports and digital control ushering the complete totalitarian police state that has been desired for decades, a reset into a dystopian reality of neo-feudalism and absolute control and hence absolute slavery. Those gene therapy drugs, with unstudied long-term effects, portend unknown side effects beyond the hundreds of thousands of people already killed and injured.

Former Pfizer VP Dr. Michael Yeadon: COVID 'vaccines' are going to kill you[215]
-April 18, 2021

---

[214] https://brandnewtube.com/watch/why-and-how-they-plan-to-kill-seven-billion_loR7dirywg1993R.html
https://www.youtube.com/watch?v=-tiqoH1iKG0
https://articles.mercola.com/sites/articles/archive/2021/05/15/planet-lockdown.aspx?ui=152220df1deda081f73727bc10a8407027b248ba493a7ce71f4a1e73a6c1d882&sd=20200829&cid_source=dnl&cid_medium=email&cid_content=art1HL&cid=20210515&mid=DM885052&rid=1158339911
[215] https://prn.fm/progressive-commentary-hour-04-28-21/

The global deep state: A new world order brought to you by COVID-19[216]

Published Wednesday, Apr. 28, 2021
By John W. Whitehead & Nisha Whitehead

Many credentialed persons in the health field have been coming forward expressing alarm and calling for a halt of the experimental mass gene therapy injections (referred to as "vaccines") due to previously unthinkable effects on humanity itself. Among others, Dr. Vanden Bossche and Dr. Michael Yeadon, Dr. Sherri Tenpenny, and Dr. Lawrence B. Palevsky[217] warn of the possible dangers, of instituting a mass injection program with unproven benefits and unknown long-term side effects, including vaccine escape and possible irreversible genetic changes as well as a possible danger to unvaccinated persons; some dangers could lead to the extinction of the human race. Therefore, just as the dangers, of exploding a nuclear weapon in 1945, including the possible incineration of the entire atmosphere of planet earth, were ignored, so too the possible dangers of mass injections with unknown, unstudied gene therapies have been ignored. The same types of personalities, the sociopathic politicians and corporatists, along with the "narcissistic scientist intellectual personality disorder" suffering scientists, who think their hubristic mechanical theories, about biological organisms, cannot be wrong because in their skewed minds their theories represent correct and complete knowledge.

Specifically, in the context of how scientific intellectuals or technocratic personalities, in general, many, not all, see their positions in society, often from a "narcissistic scientist intellectual personality disorder" perspective. For the purpose of this book, the reference to "narcissistic scientist intellectual personality disorder" is a term coined to encapsulate the idea that many scientists (in medical, engineering, physics, etc. disciplines) have that is based on the idea that since they think about things scientifically, and

---

[216] https://augustafreepress.com/the-global-deep-state-a-new-world-order-brought-to-you-by-covid-19/
[217] https://thedailycoin.org/2021/04/26/critically-thinking-with-dr-sherri-tenpenny-dr-lawrence-b-palevsky-video/
https://www.bitchute.com/video/4Bb4KAJ4kppw/

have done scientific studies, etc. that they are, therefore, correct in their assessments and or theories (proven or unproven). Furthermore, since they are correct and anyone else who thinks about things in different ways cannot possibly arrive at truth and therefore they have the right to dictate policies related to scientific issues over personal sovereignty and individual human rights. That hubris means that anyone else who questions them or proposes other theories or answers to issues of life is to be dismissed and now ridiculed, canceled and threatened with loss of income. Thinking that complex systems of nature and the human body can be understood with the mind, the intellect and theories, models and concepts alone and treating these theories, which can only be composed of partial information, as facts or absolute truth may be considered as a delusion. This narcissistic scientist intellectual personality disorder plays into the hands of power elite personalities, who use the scientists as front groups to impose varied social engineering policies that even the narcissistic scientist intellectual personality disorder suffering scientists may not be aware of or may not even care about. To the aforesaid we may add any of the regular human failings including greed, lust for prestige, complexes and psychological issues suffered by many humans.

They thereby forge ahead without considering the consequences of their actions and blind themselves to those consequences by citing an imagined virtue of "science for science's sake". These are the same people, who, without care over the side effects of 2G, 3G, and 4G technology are now implementing 5G technology, the skewed intellect scientists, sociopathic greedy corporatists, and corrupt politicians along with armies of technicians in telecommunication companies, who just want a paycheck and not think of any consequences of their actions. These sectors of humanity coupled with the masses of ignorant followers, who defer to the sociopaths and mentally defective scientists the right to control medical science and public health are the sources the pose as much of a threat to humanity as the sociopaths and mentally damaged scientists who created nuclear weapons and instituted the cold war which they are constantly trying to restart.

R. F. Kennedy Jr. warns: Don't take a COVID-19 vaccine under any circumstances[218]

---

[218] https://blogfactory.co.uk/2021/02/08/kennedy-jr-warns-dont-take-a-covid-19-vaccine-under-any-circumstances/

From Barbarians to Snowflakes: Sociopathy, Fragility, Fear and Social Degradation.

This volume does not purport to say that all persons in society are either pathological. Sociopathic, fragile, deluded, or degraded. It is, however, the message that the driving force in society is captured by those negative streams of thought and desire. That is to say, while not all members of the society are sociopathic as their leaders, nevertheless, the society is captured by the sociopathic ideologies and impetuses that have, as their outcomes, sociopathic values and actions by the society as a whole.

The degraded state of society, as a whole, is compounded with the advent of pathological fragility[219] in many members of the society. The development of the society descending into ethical and political degradation accelerating faster than previous decades, may be traced to the presidency of Ronal Reagan with the October Surprise corrupt presidential win in the year 1980, and followed by a string of corruptions up to the Iran-Contra scandal. The degradation of USA and western society accelerated further, with the sharp downturn in politics with the first gulf war and the democratic party capitulation to corporate powers, ushered in by president Bill Clinton. Then the degradation accelerated further with development of the internet and the European Union in the mid to late-1990s. The degradation of the democratic party was paired with the descent of the republican party.

The Republican Revolution '94, also known as the Gingrich Revolution, refers to the Republican Party electoral success in the 1994 U.S. midterm elections. Those elections resulted in a net gain of 54 seats in the House of Representatives, and a pickup of eight seats in the Senate, giving the republican party solid control of congress. This victory occurred under the auspices of republican party operatives such as Newt Gingrich who, along with others, exacerbated the preexisting unethical nature of politics, taking it to the level of open acrimony, mudslinging, and do or say anything, including truth or bald-faced lies, be they to destroy an opponent or the country, to achieve political victory. In this context, the actions of Gingrich and his republican cohorts were an open return, without the pretense of civility or manners, to barbarism and barbarian culture. This brand of open acrimonious, spiteful, hostile, and ill-willed relating quickly spread among the rank and file party followers and also affected their opponents, the democratic party, who today have moved from liberalism (tolerance, equal

---

[219] https://prn.fm/gary-null-show-05-06-21/

rights, free speech advocates) to neo-liberalism (corporatist agenda, censorship, totalitarianism, and imperialism) seek to brand republicans as anti-American, traitors, etc. and censor/cancel them.

On the other end of the political spectrum, the descent to open corporatism, which is another word for fascism, without pretense, was the door opened by president Clinton and his neoliberal cohorts. These dual degraded forms of politics used the fear of personal safety, real or imagined, in terms of crime, which was increasing throughout the 1970s to 1990s, as a tool for instilling fear in the population to facilitate support for the prison industrial complex and the police industrial complex. Some of the tactics used to instill that fear began in the 1980s with president Reagan and his cohorts, in the form of the constant media and political messages supporting and conflating racism with crack cocaine, the danger of black males, and the danger of child kidnappings. These fears ushered in laws such as the three-strike incarceration, and other laws, approved by Bill Clinton, that increased the prison population of the USA to the highest in the world. This also created a fear-mongered society, ripe for tough-on-crime laws and heavy-handed police actions domestically and constant wars internationally. So the fear-mongered society develops the pathology of fragility delusion that plays into the hands of the never-ending fearmongering by the coordinated colluding (fascistic) government and media officials. Thus, the allowance of corrupt and sociopathic leaders leads to the damage of the individuals in the society that sought those leaders out as a means to allay their fears. This is like seeking out cancer to heal the body riddled with cancer.

The negative course of politics contributed to the degradation of the socialization process in the culture as the latest generation (millennials) grew up amidst the political aforesaid decay and the malfeasance and fascistic corruption of the stock market[220] that led to the doc.com crash and the fraudulent election of George W. Bush as president with his neo-conservative imperial warmongering handlers. So, the toxic social and political environment that culminated in the 1990s led to a society of low or no morals in politics, matched by low or no morals in corporations, commerce, and international affairs; in short, a descent into amorality where truth and ethics are a choice rather than a responsibility or they are a factor of personal belief, informed by personal feelings, rather than objective reviewing of facts and open impersonal discussions.

---

[220] https://www.corbettreport.com/markets/

Before the present accelerating political descent into fascism, the degradation of health in society was already in effect due to the denaturing of food caused by corporate industrial farming. Additionally, the physical and mental degradation suffered by many people, due to degradation of food from over-farming and industrial processing of food, was matched by the descent of medical "science", that was already corrupt due to its faith-based belief in the germ theory and allopathic drug theory. These degradations have facilitated the corrupt leaders' movement towards medical tyranny that has now degraded the health of the population further and foisted experimental genetic modified food and chemical gene therapies and chemical dependencies, on the society. The chemical dependences foisted on the population by supposedly legitimate drug companies and health workers far exceeds the drug addictions, loss of physical and mental health, loss of productive work time and deaths due to outlaw drug cartels. The aforesaid is exacerbated by the relentless corporate quest for profits regardless of the degradation to the environment. The corporate pollution is compounded by the proven geoengineering jet spraying that contains aluminum, barium, and other chemicals purportedly to stem global warming but which also have the effect of causing diseases such as cancer and alzheimer's.[221] With the above-mentioned issues coupled with the descent into amorality, society develops into an unhinged, dull, animal instinct-driven culture. In such a culture people are driven exclusively by feelings and thus are easily manipulated by charlatans, and sociopaths, who themselves are ignorant, fear-driven, control and power-obsessed personalities incapable of rational thought with empathy or concern for the well-being of society, their own wellbeing or the wellbeing of their own progeny.

These issues, coupled, with the advent of social media in the late 2000s produced a generation of social media-addicted personalities who derive their sense of wellbeing from clicks on a phone screen instead of human interaction, rational thought, and non-traumatized feelings. They are as if fragile persons, who because of their pathology of fragility, have bought into and have fed into and support the present day cancel culture; in other words, their pathology supports and exacerbates their pathology in support of the power elite police state agenda. This generation of fragile persons complains when anything does not meet their expectations, complains when teachers challenge them, complains when they do not get the grade they think they should have, whether they earned it or not, and shout down any

---

[221] https://prn.fm/gary-null-show-05-06-21/

speaker on campus that does not conform to their thoughts and opinions about reality. This generation of fragile persons has been referred to as the "safe space and snowflake generation" since most any issue of substance, affecting their lives, in reality or imagined, causes "existential" fear in them requiring them to seek a safe place away from the stressor, the offending situation or ideas. The appearance is that they, as if, like little snowflakes that disintegrate at the slightest touch, must seek safety or must, by any means, stop or cancel, the issue, item, or person that they find threatening to their very existence.

From a Maat Philosophy perspective, the outcome of a society containing many fragile personalities could be seen as the inevitable result of a society not led and governed by people with an authentic ethical conscience. Thus, the lack of ethics in the society, due to the corrosive outcomes of fascist capitalist and sociopathic leadership over decades, has led to the current and increasing degradation of society that is now, supported by its own damaged, miseducated, misled, fear-mongered and corrupted population, arriving at a full-on *neo-feudal fascist, totalitarian, surveillance police state*.

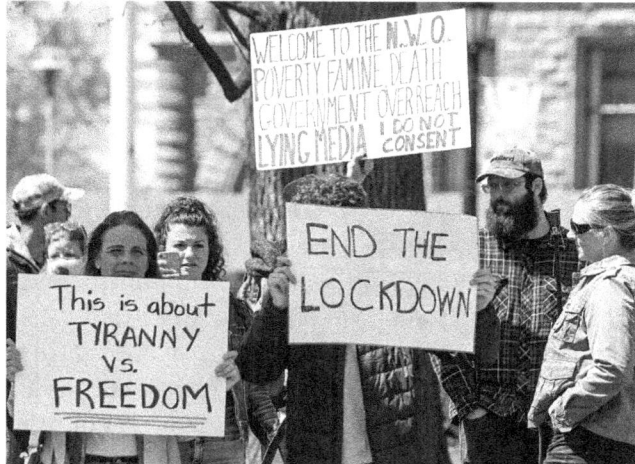

An anti-lockdown protest in front of the Ontario Legislative Building in Queen's Park, Toronto, April 25, 2020

THE BANE OF HUMANITY AND THE ANSWER FROM ETHIOCRACY

THE FAILURE OF THE US CONSTITUTION AND THE DELUSION OF THE FOUNDING FATHERS

The so-called Founding Fathers of the United States constitution recognized that ordinary human beings were ill equipped to run their own affairs as a society. They also recognized the problems of monarchy. So, they set out to create a system of government that checks the powers of the aristocracy and prevents power from getting into the hands of ordinary citizens. However, they failed to account for the possibility of the aristocracy developing into an oligarchic plutocratic class that would subvert every aspect of the social institutions. This means that the supposed elites of the population are just as ill equipped to carry on a society that promotes wellbeing for all of its members. Both groups suffer from the vicissitudes of the immature and egoistically corrupt human personality. Thus, the ideals of any system of government are subject to failure if the people managing the implementations of those ideals are themselves flawed, corrupt individuals. Therefore, neither group can be entrusted with those ideals, as leaders.

ANCIENT EGYPTIAN WISDOM OF SECULAR GOVERNMENT[222]

In Ancient Egypt neither group was given authority over the society. Instead, a group of men and women who were dedicated to the study and implementation of MAAT wisdom were entrusted with the management of every aspect of society. This form of government has been termed "**ethiocracy**." (ethical-government or government rule by ethics and ethical persons). This trust rewarded Ancient Egyptian society with thousands of years of social equity, including gender equality that allowed the society to prosper longer than any other society in human history. Those men and women were priests and priestesses who sought to establish themselves on the wisdom of Maat Philosophy and apply that wisdom in secular and non-secular life. It was that guidance that allowed them to equitably manage the sometimes turbulent waters of human life and provide

---

[222] See the book *Ancient Egyptian Economics* by Dr. Muata Ashby

a viable and sustainable venue for human life that did not diminish the environmental capacity to sustain life for future generations.

PERSONAL SOVEREIGNTY AS A FOUNDATION FOR SECULAR SOCIAL BALANCE AND PROSPERITY AND SPIRITUAL ENLIGHTENMENT

This book has introduced the issue of personal sovereignty as a primary necessity especially in a time where kakistocracy rules over nations worldwide. In ancient times, when the society was ruled by those who were indeed worthy of trust (society such as Ancient Egypt), due to their life of ethical conscience, the decision to entrust one's wellbeing to such a principled group would be justified. However, even that trust should be well considered, without duress or coercion. Therefore, the assertion of personal sovereignty cannot be un-asserted even in a positive or agreeable situation. In agreeable or disagreeable situations alike, the personal sovereignty is to be asserted because only that way is it possible to prevent falling into the delusion of safety and security in life, which no one can provide. The assertion of personal sovereignty causes a personality to maintain self-awareness aside from the personal desires or delusions of others. Thus, in order to promote the best possible situation in life, the decisions in life should be made with informed consent and with un-coerced volition. Through this assertion of personal sovereignty, an individual is best able to maintain sanity (grasp on truth) and not fall into delusions that would be damaging to themselves and to the society as a whole. Then that personal sovereignty is able to blossom into higher forms of self-awareness growing to universal spiritual awareness as the self being more than the individual ego but rather the universal essential being of Creation (spiritual enlightenment). That spiritual enlightenment, experienced by the practitioners of Maat wisdom, empowers the secular application of their ethics as those in charge of society because they are living and sharing their notions of ethical conscience through their actions of which Maat wisdom, in social policy, is the resulting application in the real world. Otherwise, the person who give up personal sovereignty can become the object of theirs and other's delusions and a prisoner of the delusion of a society that is locked up in the delusion of its own hubristic existence.

CONCLUSION: A SPIRITUAL APPEAL FROM ANCIENT EGYPTIAN MAAT WISDOM

Going forward, the duty of a mature human being is to develop critical thinking skills and make the best-informed decisions to protect health and promote wellbeing. The questions that should be asked are why are there so many of the masses so degraded in terms of intelligence, knowledge, and critical thinking skills? Why are such mentally damaged, deranged and psychotic individuals, the skewed intellectual personality disorder suffering scientists, the sociopathic greedy corporatists, and corrupt politicians along with armies of technicians allowed to control and direct the course of humanity? If they are a danger to humanity is it not up to humanity to remove these personalities as one would remove a metastasized cancer? If they have been and are being allowed to maintain their posts and spew their propaganda, spew toxic pollutions with their industries and impose chemical therapies, is not humanity itself to blame for its own suffering or even demise? These rhetorical questions call for righteous indignation followed by righteous action in response to the failure of humanity to live up to its own needs instead of ceding the rights and sovereignty of the human being to sociopaths and psychotic individuals. What actions can be and should be taken now and going forward? First, there must be action to inform oneself of truth based on verifiable facts. No longer is it viable to have a society where people can be allowed to live by their opinions and make up their own facts, instead of a society that agrees to objective verifiable facts. Of course, the media cannot be allowed to spew the toxic messages based on political expediency as opposed to ethical and factual findings. Also, importantly, science cannot be allowed to become corrupted by greedy scientists, billionaires, and politicians. Perhaps most important, no cause is sufficient to abrogate peoples human rights even if there is a pandemic; so medical tyranny is unacceptable. Then there needs to be bolstering of one's own capacity to live by those truths. The capacity to live by truth is built on physical and mental health, spiritual strength and ethics, living with the ideal of right action. The "Spiritual Appeal" is a possible pathway for finding and growing spiritual strength, ethical and moral fortitude, and indomitable capacity for living as an ethically conscious individual, a mature and powerful human being who can counter the forces of ignorance and sociopathy and succeed in the struggle of life, to promote physical, mental and spiritual health for all.

Unlike the "Fear Appeal" weapon of the power elite, the "Spiritual Appeal" is an appeal to that part of human existence that calls upon the higher nature of a human being that is beyond worldly fear and thus is more powerful than worldly fears that come from life situations including disasters, calamities, personal loss, and confrontation with inimical personalities that mean one harm. According to Ancient Egyptian MAAT wisdom, the highest truth is discovering and allowing one's higher nature (Zokar – image above) to rule over one's personality instead of allowing ignorance, fear and egoism to control one's life.

Verse 10.

10.1. *puy en Zokar user-f auu aah [send] im ren f*
10.2. that of King of Netherworld almighty he expansion great [fear] in name his
10.3. ...(contextual translation)

> That one: *Zokar* which means "sovereign of the netherworld plane of existence;" the soul that is master of the personality. In this capacity he is almighty and his essence spreads expansively, so much so as to cause awe, admiration, and awestricken feelings; this all occurs when a person recognizes their existence in his name...[223]

When ignorance, fear and egoism control one's life, this is the degraded aspect of the personality that can be affected by inimical forces and through which fear arises due to ignorance and the egoistic desires to protect comforts, convenience and or perceived wealth or well-being in the short-run while ignoring, practicing willful ignorance or being unmindful about the total loss of freedom, safety, security and well-being, that occurs in the longer run. When one's sovereign soul-self (Zokar) rules over one's life one will not be as susceptible to charlatans, demagogues, or predator elite personalities of the world. When one's soul rules over one's life one is not interested in hoarding or partisanship but rather in the well-being of all which requires cooperation based on a common goal of seeking,

---

[223] Translation by Dr. Muata Ashby

understanding and living by truth and not by lies and fears. This is the internecine conflict between maat (truth) and fascism. Maat wisdom is about the truth of universal humanity and therefore demands ethical caring for the well-being of all humanity and nature based on the common spiritual bond that all souls have, while fascism is about the egoistic pursuit of segregation, commodification, and exploitation of people for sociopathic ends. Living one's existence in the name of one's higher self, one's immortal soul, Zokar has the effect of allowing one to live with dignity and power that strikes fear in the unrighteous instead of living in fear which is the delight of the predator class, the global power elite. Maat means truth and the conflict of Maat vs Fascism and the police state is a war of good vs evil and now a war between truth vs deception, the search for truth vs censorship and cancel culture. Truth wins, in the end, because truth is reality and falsehood is an illusory, and therefore, insubstantial façade of the unrighteous personality. Therefore, those who pursue truth inevitably discover it, while those who promote distortion, lies and deception as well as those who follow them, will remain in the delusion of the deception until the suffering from the delusion is too much to bear.[224]

THE AUSTERITY OF MAAT MEANS...

Before the year 2020 only some members of the population (the poor, the purposely dispossessed, discriminated against, or ostracized) were experiencing full adverse conditions; some experienced adversity some of the time. But now it would seem that all of the members of the underclasses (classes below the power elite and technocratic bureaucracy) are experiencing severe adversity in terms of psychological and or physical stress and distress. Such times as the challenges that are posed by the segment of the population that seeks totalitarian control, may be understood as a time of adversity. In a time of adversity, it is necessary to take an austere posture, physically, mentally, and spiritually.

Austerity means recognizing that the time of acting as if everything is fine, the wishful thinking that the world always goes on as before or good times are around the corner just as soon as everyone sees the truth or as soon as we vote in a "good guy" or as soon as everybody acquiesces to wear a mask and takes the vaccine without question, are delusions. ***Austerity means***

---

[224] https://brandnewtube.com/v/tZ5Cbn

recognizing that the political and power elite classes are not knights in shining armor desiring to save anyone but empower themselves. *Austerity means* taking stock of what is real and not following delusions. *Austerity means* looking within oneself and developing the resources to weather the storm of social, political, and economic strife. *Austerity means* looking to the inner spirit instead of external possessions or personalities, for comfort and fulfillment. *Austerity means* not just paying lip service to one's maatian ethical conscience and sharing that with those who are also similarly seeking to find physical, mental, and spiritual health, which are the pathways to political, economic freedom and prosperity, and spiritual emancipation. Maat ethics are a reflection of spiritual insight. Therefore, maatian ethical study and practice is the opening up of spiritual evolution that surpasses worldly situations and histories. Therefore, this current adverse period in history, is an opportunity to practice austerity that helps us turn towards our spiritual source so as to discover inner peace and the clarity to promote social and political peace. Austerity can be a concerted effort to take time for reflection and considered thought about the past instead of constantly moving forward, being reactionary and unmindful being more susceptible to the traps of personal and societal egoism, desires and delusion that are preyed upon by the power elite, the greedy, the con-artists and the charlatans of humanity. In this way, the adversity can be turned to austerity and the austerity to spiritual evolution, spiritual power that wins out over ignorance, immorality, amorality, sociopathy and evil.

MAAT: Ancient Egyptian Goddess of Truth and Ethical Conscience

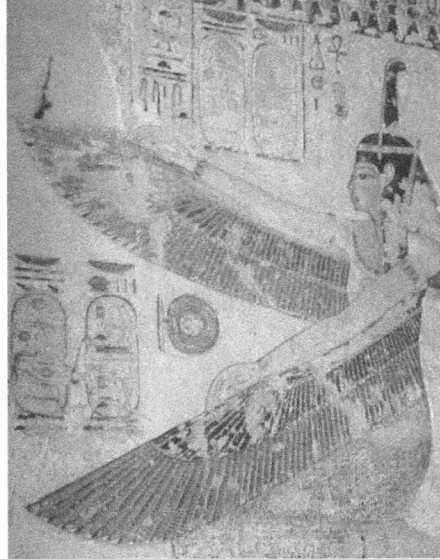

Ancient Egyptian Maat Wisdom:

"When emotions are society's objective, tyranny will govern regardless of the ruling class."

Maat Philosophy is based on the legacy of Ancient Egyptian priests and priestesses that led to the creation and sustainability of a civilization that persisted for thousands of years. Maat philosophy, the wisdom of righteousness, order, and truth, involves a lifestyle that promotes the health of body and mind; it is a discipline of living, thinking, and feeling by truth as opposed to the whims or vicissitudes of the changeable personality.

Maat Philosophy involves the study of ethical conscience and its effects on the personality and its importance for building viable and sustainable politics for creating righteous social, political, and economic institutions leading to general justice, health and prosperity for the whole society. It necessarily relates to gaining insight into the nature of life and the spiritual origins of Creation. In that insight, the will, feeling, and understanding of their place in Creation and their kinship of humanity and Creation becomes clarified such that a human being can realize the impetus of non-violence and harmonization with life. Those proprieties are counter to the need for the acquisition of inordinate wealth or the acquisition of power. It also precludes the need for social imbalances and the capacity for sociopathic or mentally diseased, or spiritually deficient personalities to be in positions that could negatively affect the population, just as any other personality exhibiting deviance from that which is, again, the wisdom of righteousness, order, and truth, a lifestyle that promotes the health of body and mind, living, thinking and feeling by truth, etc.

In this context, Maat Philosophy promotes that which affirms truth and supports life and conversely discourages that which promotes untruth and supports death, regardless of the gain that it might seem to offer society or an individual in the short-term. A society that is not prepared to live by Maat or a similar wisdom of ethical conscience will inevitably experience instability and the vulnerability to the base feelings and desires of the population generally and the direst effects from the emergence, in such a society that would allow it, of the kakistocracy that would lead to fascism and police state politics and cultures. For more on Maat Philosophy, and to start the movement towards personal, societal freedom from the kakistocracy of fascism and the police state, and to move towards personal, spiritual empowerment and enlightenment, see the book *INTRODUCTION TO MAAT PHILOSOPHY* by Dr. Muat Ashby (www.egyptianyogabooks.com).

Steps to Learning about and Living By Maat Philosophy

Now, in early 2021 the USA does have a totalitarian government and a police state in the ascendency. How long will this continue and to what extent will it develop? How many people will suffer before, if and when the fascist totalitarian surveillance police state that is the USA government and economy will be realized as a vacuous, evil project and revolted against by the population or collapses, under the weight of its own degradation, into the chaos of political and social mayhem of mobocracy or ochlocracy or complete neo-feudalism? The answers to those questions are uncertain. In the meantime, it is up to the reader to make sense of the situation, protect their lives and work towards living a life of truth, and if possible, cooperating with others of like mind to forge a path of ethical and environmentally sustainable life, a path seeking to follow MAAT (truth-ethical conscience and spiritual awareness that recognizes the sanctity and sovereignty of all human beings), regardless of what the future may hold. It is necessary to avoid (opt-out of) participating in and or collaborating with those who are irrational, unethical, or corrupt, as much as possible. It is necessary to avoid, as much as possible, being on the surveillance grid, participating in the agenda to globally centralize authority over human rights (i.e. civil liberties, free speech, free will, freedom of movement, privacy, personal bodily sovereignty), dictating where, when, how people must live and interact, by people who are unelected corporate bureaucrats.

It means avoiding the smart devices, smart cities, digital currencies, corrupt media, and social media traps whereby one exposes one's personal information and where by mere participation one is exposing oneself to surveillance, commodification, and subliminal psychological manipulation. It means rejecting slogans like "the new normal" being imposed by unelected power elite supra-governmental institutions using scientific lies and political made up mandates such as those used to justify mask-wearing, social distancing, and lockdowns; it means working with those of like mind to assert independence from the autocratic police state and to affirm one's humanity, sovereignty, intellect, and ethical nature.

If some of the reflections and objectives discussed in this volume are to be pursued, it is recommended to look for geographical areas with less human population density and less of a chance of mandating vaccines, with fewer numbers of reactionary and unmindful people and instead look for areas with more progressive personalities, with more populations willing to apply critical thinking, protect innate human rights and apply ethical conscience instead of proximity to populations living in fearful lockstep and cooperating with sociopathic and criminal leaders.

It is recommended to consider forming small groups to cooperate with or perhaps joining with. Take time to study Maat philosophy, pursue, understand and uphold truth in life instead of living out of pleasure-seeking and sheepish ignorant following of con artists, charlatans, demagogues, and sociopaths, be they in one's own family, community, spiritual organizations, corporations, or politics. Some resources include:[225]

---

[225] Resources for maat vs fascism
https://prn.fm/gary-null-show-01-18-21/
https://prn.fm/gary-null-show-01-21-21/
https://prn.fm/gary-null-show-01-19-21/
https://www.youtube.com/watch?v=XtChmdp_ktI
https://www.youtube.com/watch?v=dZuLEvfLNyU&t=872s
https://www.youtube.com/watch?v=qjmzfYquaa8
https://youtu.be/bHwcQQbLuCw

Book: Introduction to MAAT PHILOSOPHY
https://www.egyptianyogabooks.com/
www.egyptianmysteries.org,
https://www.itmtrading.com/blog/lynette-zang-interviews/
www.ic.org,
www.freedomcells.org,
www.thegreaterreset.org,
www.makeamericansfreeagain.com,
www.standforhealthfreedom.com

Finally, while engaging in efforts to counter fascism and the police state, on ethical grounds, also make an effort not to support fascism and the police state by participating in social media, mainstream media or believing the lies of those who have proven their duplicity and corruption (politicians, health officials, corporations, etc. Additionally, opt-out, do not cooperate with their efforts or with those who support them. So do not support businesses that support lockdowns and forced vaccines. This may mean not supporting schools or any other institutions that are going along with the lies, unethical fascism and the police state agendas. By asserting one's humanity, personal sovereignty and spiritual nature, and not supporting fascism and the police state one is automatically reducing their power and increasing one's own as one joins together with others, of like mind, to collectively increase strength to uphold ethics and justice for oneself and for posterity. In so doing, one promotes one's spiritual evolution while enhancing the capacity for all life to continue, as nature intended, providing a venue for experiencing the magnanimity and glorious nature of the Divine manifesting as all Creation.

HTP

---

https://www.youtube.com/watch?v=bVPSdVp0FiM&t=3001s

INDEX

Absolute, 191
Africa, 8, 9, 137, 197, 204, 206, 208
African American, 88, 125
African Proverbial Wisdom Teachings, 213
African Religion, 191, 199, 203
Alexander The Great, 143
Allopathic, 192
Amen, 12
Amenta, 198
Amentet, 200
American Dream, 127
American Heritage Dictionary, Dictionary, 203
American Theocracy, 207
American way of life, 97
Americas, 59
Ancient Egypt, 8, 9, 13, 19, 87, 95, 120, 178, 179, 182, 191, 192, 193, 194, 195, 196, 197, 198, 199, 200, 201, 202, 203, 204, 205, 206, 207, 208, 211, 212, 213, 214, 215, 216, 217
Ancient Egyptian Wisdom Texts, 8, 212
anger, 53, 56, 92, 102, 143, 148, 202
anti-American, 111, 173
Anu, 199
Anu (Greek Heliopolis), 199
Anunian Theology, 199
Aryan, 193
Asar, 197, 198, 200, 201
Asar and Aset, 197
Asarian Resurrection, 197, 201, 202, 204
Aset, 11, 194, 197, 198, 200, 201
Aset (Isis), 11, 194, 197, 198, 200, 201

Ashanti, 213
Asia, 208
Asia Minor, 208
Asiatic, 206, 208
Assyrians, 211
Astral, 198
Astral Plane, 198
Atlantis, 205
Attila, 143
Austerity, 180
Awakening, 197, 216
Barbarians, 172
Bas, 150
Being, 8, 12, 200
Bhagavad Gita, 211
Bible, 200, 201
bin Laden, Osama, 125
Black, 150, 151, 208
Black Africa, 208
black people, 88
Body, 216
Bolivia, 111
Book of Coming Forth By Day, 11, 198
Book of the Dead, see also Rau Nu Prt M Hru, 199, 212
British empire, 143
Buddha, 204, 206, 218
Buddhism, 199, 206
Buddhist, 197, 206
Bush, George W., 89, 124, 173
Canada, 119, 134
Cancer, 30, 84
Capitalism, 117, 118, 120, 121
capitalist system, 27
Carter, Jimmy, 100
Catholic, 200
Catholic Church, 200
ceaseless-ness and regularity, 10, 12
celebrities, 26, 45

Central Intelligence Agency, 107
Change, 71, 150
Child, 201
China, 85, 133, 134, 155, 159
Chomsky, Noam, 123
Christ, 198
Christianity, 191, 199, 200
Church, 107, 200
CIA, 107, 111, 112, 125, 134, 148, 155
civil liberties, 157, 184
civil rights, 60
Civilization, 62, 109, 194, 206, 207, 208, 215, 216
Class, ruling class, 7, 87, 94, 113, 148, 182
Clinton, Bill, 25, 102, 172, 173
CNN, 52
CNN – news reports, 52
coercion, 52, 53, 58, 61, 67, 103, 115, 126, 131, 144, 146, 207
Collapse, 62, 207, 215, 217
colonialism, 91, 134
color, 93, 130, 167, 210, 212
Color, 210
Company of gods and goddesses, 10
Conflict, 207, 213
Confucianism, 9
Congress, 2
Conscience, 182
Consciousness, 197, 212
Consciousness, human, 191
Constitution, 124
contentment, 218
Coptic, 198
cosmic force, 8, 200, 205
Cosmos, 8
Coup d'état, 157
Creation, 11, 87, 182, 197, 199, 212
Crime, 46

Culture, 8, 196, 205, 209, 216, 217
Davos, Party of, 155
Death, 67, 82, 207, 215
December, 200
delusion, 25, 26, 50, 51, 52, 55, 57, 59, 83, 85, 87, 88, 89, 90, 93, 97, 99, 100, 128, 131, 173, 181
Democratic Party, 132
Denderah, 198
depression, 14, 15, 136
Depression, 14, 136
Desire, 213
Devotional Love, 195
Diet, 192
discrimination, 88
Disease, 85
dissent,, 22, 159
Dollar, U.S. Dollar, 160, 217
Dream, 127
Dream, REM sleep, 127
drug companies, 65, 66, 114
Drugs, 30
Duat, 198
Edfu, 198
Egyptian Book of Coming Forth By Day, 198
Egyptian Mysteries, 193, 202, 203, 213, 214, 215
Egyptian Physics, 199
Egyptian Proverb, 195
EGYPTIAN PROVERBS, 195
Egyptian Yoga, 191, 193, 197, 198
Egyptian Yoga see also Kamitan Yoga, 191, 193, 197, 198, 218
Egyptologists, 203, 211
Empire culture, 207
Enlightenment, 191, 193, 194, 195, 196, 197, 199, 200, 202, 206, 213, 215, 216
ETHICS, 193, 194, 206, 207, 208, 213
Ethiopia, 213
Eucharist, 198
Europe, 115, 119, 157
evil, 19, 91, 143, 153, 181, 183, 202, 203
Evil, 204
Exercise, 21, 197

exploitation, 18, 30, 91, 92, 112, 128, 131, 148, 155, 156, 159, 180
Eye, 12
Eye of Ra, 12
Faith, 209
faith-based, 174
fascism, 28, 44, 45, 57, 58, 63, 87, 91, 95, 99, 100, 105, 106, 110, 118, 121, 133, 134, 135, 148, 152, 173, 174, 180, 183, 184, 185
fascist system, 94
Fear, 60, 61, 62, 67, 96, 98, 172, 179
Feather, 8
Federal Reserve Bank, 14, 63, 94, 138
Federal Reserve System, 14, 63, 94, 138
Finances, 216
Food, 72, 161
France, 147
free market, 127
free speech, 104, 112, 173, 184
frustration, 103
fundamentalists, 102
Galla, 213
Galla culture, 213
Geb, 197
Germany, 128
Ghana, 213
global economy, 207
Globalization, 207
God, 7, 8, 10, 12, 194, 195, 198, 199, 204, 210
Goddess, 10, 182, 200, 210
Goddesses, 197, 203
Gods, 12, 197, 203
gods and goddesses, 10, 12, 199, 203, 205
Gold, 138
Good, 132, 204
Gospels, 200
Great Depression, 14, 136
Greece, 9, 193, 205
Greek philosophy, 191
Greeks, 9, 211
Harmony, 11
Hate, 213
Hatha Yoga, 207, 208
Hathor, 197, 198, 200, 202, 218

Hatred, 213
Health, 47, 48, 72, 75, 80, 82, 86, 154, 192, 199
HEART, 201, 209
HEART (ALSO SEE AB, MIND, CONSCIENCE), 201, 209
Heaven, 200
Hekau, 217
Hermes, 215
Hermes (see also Djehuti, Thoth), 215
Hermetic, 214
Hermeticism, 215
Heru, 12, 198, 199, 200, 201, 204, 212
Heru (see Horus), 12, 198, 199, 200, 201, 204, 212
Hetheru, 202
Hetheru (Hetheru, Hathor), 202
Hieroglyphic, 196, 211, 215
Hieroglyphic Writing, language, 196, 211, 215
Hinduism, 199
Hindus, 203
hope, 56, 210
human rights, 24, 59, 60, 171, 178, 184
Humanity, 154, 202
Iamblichus, 211
illusion, 57, 117, 145
Image, 151
Immorality, 62
immune system, 31, 50, 59, 68, 71, 75, 82, 86, 98
immune system, immunity, 31, 50, 59, 68, 71, 75, 82, 86, 98
imperialism, 120, 173
India, 193, 194, 195, 197, 206, 207
Indian Yoga, 193
Indus, 193
Indus Valley, 193
Infection, 31
Inflation, 138
Initiate, 192
International Monetary Fund, see also I.M.F., 14
intolerance, 54, 101, 102, 129
Iran, 172
Iran-Contra scandal, 172
Iraq, 89, 167

Isis, 11, 194, 197, 198, 200, 218
Isis, See also Aset, 11, 194, 197, 198, 200, 218
Islam, 191
Japan, 137
Jesus, 198, 200, 201, 218
Jesus Christ, 198
Jim Crow, 93
Jimmy Carter, 100
Joseph, 38, 48, 67, 99, 108, 109, 114, 154
Judaism, 191
judges, 10, 11, 12
Judgment scene, Papyrus of Ani (Any), 11
Justice, 8
Kabbalah, 191
Kamit (Egypt), 203
Kamitan, 193, 205
Karma, 8, 11, 195
Kemetic, 206, 209, 214, 216, 218
Kennedy, John F. president, 161, 171
Khemn, see also ignorance, 203
King, 7, 89, 179, 201, 204
King Jr., Martin Luther, 89
King, Dr. Martin Luther, 89
Kingdom, 200
Kingdom of Heaven, 200
Kissinger, Henry, 125
Krishna, 201
Kybalion, 214, 215
Latino, 88
Learning, 183
left wing, 107, 108, 110, 122
Libya, 25, 90, 130
Life, 15, 155, 196, 204, 209, 210, 212
Life Force, 196, 197
Lord of Eternity, 7
Love, 85, 195, 218
Lower Egypt, 10, 12
M.D., 60
Maat, 1, 2, 7, 8, 9, 10, 11, 13, 14, 27, 87, 95, 175, 178, 180, 181, 182, 183, 184, 195, 200, 201, 205, 209, 212, 213, 214, 215, 216
MAAT, 195
Maat Philosophy, 1, 2, 8, 9, 175, 182, 183, 201, 205, 209, 215

MAATI, 195
Malawi, 213
Manu, 12
Manufacturing Consent, 123
martial law, 78, 155, 166, 169
Martin Luther, 89
Martin Luther King, 89
Marx, Karl, 110
Matter, 150, 151, 199
media, 15, 16, 21, 24, 25, 26, 27, 28, 29, 31, 43, 45, 47, 49, 50, 51, 52, 53, 54, 55, 56, 57, 58, 64, 67, 68, 69, 71, 74, 75, 76, 77, 79, 80, 82, 83, 85, 89, 98, 100, 103, 104, 105, 106, 107, 111, 112, 114, 115, 120, 125, 127, 128, 130, 131, 132, 143, 144, 148, 151, 152, 153, 155, 161, 162, 168, 173, 174, 178, 184, 185, 207
Media, 54, 107, 123
medical system, 21, 56, 67
Meditation, 192, 195, 196
Medu Neter, 203, 217
Memphite Theology, 199
Meskhenet, 8, 11, 195
Metaphysics, 199, 212
Middle East, 191
Mills, 18
Min, 197
Mind, 44, 216
Morales, Evo, 111
MSNBC, 102
murder, 16, 88, 119, 143
Music, 210
Mysteries, 193, 202, 203, 211, 213, 214, 215
mystical philosophy, 206, 212
Mysticism, 193, 194, 198, 199, 202, 206, 207, 208
Napoleon, 143
Nazi, 128
Neberdjer, 191
Nehast, 203
neo-colonial, 91, 134
neo-colonialism, 91, 134
neo-con, 173, 207
neo-conservative, 173
Neo-feudalism, 94, 95
Neter, 195, 198, 203, 204, 206, 211, 213, 216, 217

Neterian, 203, 204, 206, 216, 217, 218
Neterianism, 215, 216
Neteru, 203
Netherworld, 10, 179
Nigeria, 213
Nixon, Richard, 133
NSA, 100, 112, 155
Nu, 8
nuclear weapons, 171
Nut, 197
Obama, Barack, 23, 25, 90, 125, 130, 131, 155
Ohio, 42
Orion Star Constellation, 200
Orthodox, 203
Osama bin Laden, 125
Osiris, 7, 12, 197, 198, 204
out of thin air, money, 14, 23, 138
Park, 175
Patriot Act, 155
Paul, 150
Peace, 213, 215, 216
Peace (see also Hetep), 213, 215, 216
Persians, 211
PERT EM HERU, SEE ALSO BOOK OF THE DEAD, 198
Pharaoh, 216
Philae, 198
Philosophy, 1, 2, 8, 9, 10, 87, 182, 183, 191, 193, 194, 195, 198, 199, 201, 205, 206, 207, 208, 209, 215, 216
plutocrats, 106
police action, 153, 173
power elite, 13, 18, 21, 24, 26, 27, 30, 44, 51, 52, 53, 55, 56, 57, 58, 60, 61, 62, 63, 65, 66, 85, 88, 91, 92, 94, 95, 97, 98, 99, 100, 101, 102, 103, 105, 106, 108, 112, 117, 118, 119, 120, 121, 123, 124, 125, 127, 128, 131, 133, 134, 136, 138, 142, 143, 145, 147, 149, 151, 152, 153, 155, 156, 157, 159, 166, 169, 171, 174, 179, 180, 181, 184
Power elite, 133
president, 23, 24, 56, 72, 73, 74, 79, 89, 100, 102, 111,

119, 124, 125, 131, 133, 144, 155, 158, 162, 172, 173
pressure, 45, 68, 74, 82
priests and priestesses, 182, 197, 204
Priests and Priestesses, 193, 204
Progressive, 66
Propaganda, 18, 22, 30, 128
Proverbial Wisdom, 213
Psychiatrist, 63
Psychology, 199, 214
Ptah, 12, 199
Queen, 175, 204
Ra, 8, 10, 11, 12, 197
race, 18, 53, 78, 87, 88, 92, 93, 103, 170
racism, 9, 55, 87, 88, 92, 93, 102, 103, 107, 125, 149, 173, 214
Racism, 213
Reagan, Ronald, 25, 102, 127, 173
Realization, 194
Reflection, 13
Religion, 191, 194, 198, 199, 201, 203, 204, 205, 206, 207, 208, 216, 217, 218
Rennenet, 11
Republican Party, 79, 132, 172
reserve currency, 23
Resurrection, 197, 198, 200, 201, 202, 204
Righteousness, 8
RITUAL, 202
Rituals, 200
Roman, 143, 211
Romans, 9, 211
Rome, 205
Safe, 31, 47, 77
Sages, 9, 191, 197, 198, 202, 205, 218
Saints, 198, 218
Scribe, 8
Sebai, 206, 210, 214, 216
See also Ra-Hrakti, 8, 10, 11, 12, 197
Self (see Ba, soul, Spirit, Universal, Ba, Neter, Heru)., 8, 10, 12, 59, 87, 194, 196, 198, 202, 210
Self-created lifestyle, lifestyle, 57, 182, 183

Sema, 2, 204, 214, 215, 217
Set, 204
Seti I, 196
Sex, 197
sexism, 9, 55, 107, 149, 214
Sexism, 213
Shai, 11
Shedy, 192
Shetaut Neter, 198, 203, 204, 206, 213, 216, 217
Shetaut Neter See also Egyptian Religion, 198, 203, 204, 206, 213, 216, 217
Sirius, 200
skin, 93
Sky, 160
slavery, 57, 90, 93, 169, 203
society, 7, 8, 9, 11, 13, 14, 15, 16, 17, 21, 24, 26, 27, 45, 50, 52, 53, 55, 56, 58, 61, 64, 65, 87, 88, 90, 92, 93, 94, 96, 99, 100, 101, 103, 104, 105, 106, 107, 108, 112, 118, 119, 120, 121, 123, 124, 126, 128, 130, 132, 136, 138, 143, 144, 149, 152, 153, 155, 156, 157, 170, 172, 173, 174, 175, 178, 182, 183, 192, 203, 205, 209, 213, 214, 215, 217
Society, 155, 215, 217
sociopaths, 18, 26, 75, 95, 118, 122, 126, 171, 174, 178, 184
Soul, 204, 216
Spiritual discipline, 192
SPIRITUALITY, 193, 209, 216, 217, 218
Study, 31, 38, 54, 98, 100, 114, 123, 126, 151
Sublimation, 197
sun, 56
Sun, 56
Superpower, 207
Superpower Syndrome, 207
Superpower Syndrome Mandatory Conflict Complex, 207
Supreme Being, 8, 12, 200
Syria, 90, 131, 132
TANTRA, 197
TANTRA YOGA, 197
Taoism, 191

Television, 25, 129, 144
Temple, 198, 202, 216
Temple of Aset, 198
Temu, 12
terrorist, 89, 91
Texas, 114
The Absolute, 191
The Black, 208
The God, 197
The Gods, 197
Theban Theology, 191
Thebes, 191, 196
Theocracy, 207
Theology, 191, 199
Thoreau, Henry David, 130
Thoth, 7
Time, 85, 99
time and space, 203
Tobacco, 45
tolerance, 172
Tomb, 196
Tomb of Seti I, 196
transcendental reality, 203
Tree, 212
Tree of Life, 212
Triad, 191
Trinity, 198
Truth, 8, 182
Understanding, 11, 203, 215
United States of America, 207
Universal Consciousness, 197
Upanishads, 199, 211
USA, West, 14, 17, 19, 23, 52, 72, 87, 88, 89, 90, 97, 99, 100, 105, 106, 107, 108, 115, 119, 122, 126, 128, 131, 133, 137, 143, 155, 160, 167, 169, 172, 173, 183
Vedic, 193
Venezuela, 19
Vietnam, 89
Violence, 213
Wall Street, 125
wars, 25, 56, 91, 105, 130, 148, 173
Waset, 191
Wealth, Money, 216
weapons of mass destruction, 89, 167
Western, West, 7, 12
White, 215
white people, 92
Whitehead, 44, 170

Wisdom, 8, 178, 182, 195, 196, 211, 212, 213, 216
Wisdom (also see Djehuti, Aset), 8, 178, 182, 195, 196, 211, 212, 213, 216
World Ba, 155
World Ba XE "World Ba" nk, 155
World Economic Forum, 21, 150, 155, 156
World War II, 109, 207
Yoga, 191, 192, 193, 194, 197, 198, 199, 201, 204, 206, 207, 208, 218
Yoga of Devotion (see Yoga of Divine Love), 218
Yogic, 208, 214
Yoruba, 213

OTHER BOOKS FROM C M BOOKS

P.O.Box 570459
Miami, Florida, 33257
(305) 378-6253 Fax: (305) 378-6253

Prices subject to change.

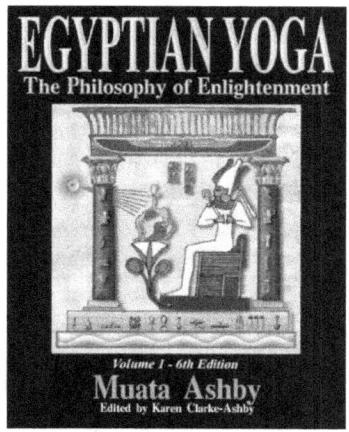

1. **EGYPTIAN YOGA: THE PHILOSOPHY OF ENLIGHTENMENT** An original, fully illustrated work, including hieroglyphs, detailing the meaning of the Egyptian mysteries, tantric yoga, psycho-spiritual and physical exercises. Egyptian Yoga is a guide to the practice of the highest spiritual philosophy which leads to absolute freedom from human misery and to immortality. It is well known by scholars that Egyptian philosophy is the basis of Western and Middle Eastern religious philosophies such as *Christianity*, *Islam*, *Judaism*, the *Kabala*, and Greek philosophy, but what about Indian philosophy, Yoga and Taoism? What were the original teachings? How can they be practiced today? What is the source of pain and suffering in the world and what is the solution? Discover the deepest mysteries of the mind and universe within and outside of yourself. 8.5" X 11" ISBN: 1-884564-01-1 Soft $19.95

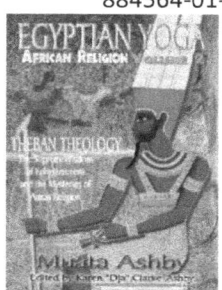

2. *EGYPTIAN YOGA: African Religion Volume 2- Theban Theology U.S.* In this long awaited sequel to *Egyptian Yoga: The Philosophy of Enlightenment* you will take a fascinating and enlightening journey back in time and discover the teachings which constituted the epitome of Ancient Egyptian spiritual wisdom. What are the disciplines which lead to the fulfillment of all desires? Delve into the three states of consciousness (waking, dream and deep sleep) and the fourth state which transcends them all, Neberdjer, "The Absolute." These teachings of the city of Waste (Thebes) were the crowning achievement of the Sages of Ancient Egypt. They establish the standard mystical keys for understanding the profound mystical symbolism of the Triad of human consciousness. ISBN 1-884564-39-9 $23.95

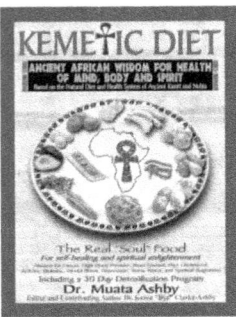

3. **THE KEMETIC DIET: GUIDE TO HEALTH, DIET AND FASTING** Health issues have always been important to human beings since the beginning of time. The earliest records of history show that the art of healing was held in high esteem since the time of Ancient Egypt. In the early 20th century, medical doctors had almost attained the status of sainthood by the promotion of the idea that they alone were "scientists" while other healing modalities and traditional healers who did not follow the "scientific method' were nothing but superstitious, ignorant charlatans who at best would take the money of their clients and at worst kill them with the unscientific "snake oils" and "irrational theories". In the late 20th century, the failure of the modern medical establishment's ability to lead the general public to good health, promoted the move by many in society towards "alternative medicine". Alternative medicine disciplines are those healing modalities which do not adhere to the philosophy of allopathic medicine. Allopathic medicine is what medical doctors practice by an large. It is the theory that disease is caused by agencies outside the body such as bacteria, viruses or physical means which affect the body. These can therefore be treated by medicines and therapies The natural healing method began in the absence of extensive technologies with the idea that all the answers for health may be found in nature or rather, the deviation from nature. Therefore, the health of the body can be restored by correcting the aberration and thereby restoring balance. This is the area that will be covered in this volume. Allopathic techniques have their place in the art of healing. However, we should not forget that the body is a grand achievement of the spirit and built into it is the capacity to maintain itself and heal itself. Ashby, Muata ISBN: 1-884564-49-6 $28.95

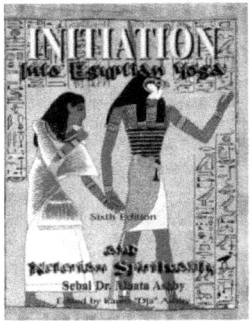

4. **INITIATION INTO EGYPTIAN YOGA** Shedy: Spiritual discipline or program, to go deeply into the mysteries, to study the mystery teachings and literature profoundly, to penetrate the mysteries. You will learn about the mysteries of initiation into the teachings and practice of Yoga and how to become an Initiate of the mystical sciences. This insightful manual is the first in a series which introduces you to the goals of daily spiritual and yoga practices: Meditation, Diet, Words of Power and the ancient wisdom teachings. 8.5" X 11" ISBN 1-884564-02-X Soft Cover $24.95 U.S.

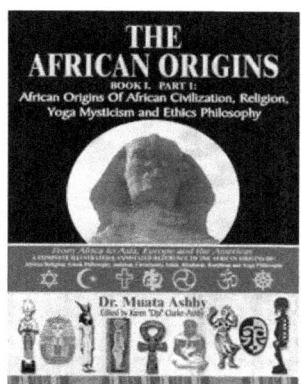

5. THE AFRICAN ORIGINS OF CIVILIZATION, RELIGION AND YOGA SPIRITUALITY AND ETHICS PHILOSOPHY HARD COVER EDITION Part 1, Part 2, Part 3 in one volume 683 Pages Hard Cover First Edition Three volumes in one. Over the past several years I have been asked to put together in one volume the most important evidences showing the correlations and common teachings between Kami tan (Ancient Egyptian) culture and religion and that of India. The questions of the history of Ancient Egypt, and the latest archeological evidences showing civilization and culture in Ancient Egypt and its spread to other countries, has intrigued many scholars as well as mystics over the years. Also, the possibility that Ancient Egyptian Priests and Priestesses migrated to Greece, India and other countries to carry on the traditions of the Ancient Egyptian Mysteries, has been speculated over the years as well. In chapter 1 of the book *Egyptian Yoga The Philosophy of Enlightenment*, 1995, I first introduced the deepest comparison between Ancient Egypt and India that had been brought forth up to that time. Now, in the year 2001 this new book, THE AFRICAN ORIGINS OF CIVILIZATION, MYSTICAL RELIGION AND YOGA PHILOSOPHY, more fully explores the motifs, symbols and philosophical correlations between Ancient Egyptian and Indian mysticism and clearly shows not only that Ancient Egypt and India were connected culturally but also spiritually. How does this knowledge help the spiritual aspirant? This discovery has great importance for the Yogis and mystics who follow the philosophy of Ancient Egypt and the mysticism of India. It means that India has a longer history and heritage than was previously understood. It shows that the mysteries of Ancient Egypt were essentially a yoga tradition which did not die but rather developed into the modern day systems of Yoga technology of India. It further shows that African culture developed Yoga Mysticism earlier than any other civilization in history. All of this expands our understanding of the unity of culture and the deep legacy of Yoga, which stretches into the distant past, beyond the Indus Valley civilization, the earliest known high culture in India as well as the Vedic tradition of Aryan culture. Therefore, Yoga culture and mysticism is the oldest known tradition of spiritual development and Indian mysticism is an extension of the Ancient Egyptian mysticism. By understanding the legacy which Ancient Egypt gave to India the mysticism of India is better understood and by comprehending the heritage of Indian Yoga, which is rooted in Ancient Egypt the Mysticism of Ancient Egypt is also better understood. This expanded understanding allows us to prove the underlying kinship of humanity, through the common symbols,

motifs and philosophies which are not disparate and confusing teachings but in reality expressions of the same study of truth through metaphysics and mystical realization of Self. (HARD COVER) ISBN: 1-884564-50-X $45.00 U.S. 81/2" X 11"

6. *AFRICAN ORIGINS BOOK 1 PART 1* African Origins of African Civilization, Religion, Yoga Mysticism and Ethics Philosophy- Soft Cover $24.95 ISBN: 1-884564-55-0

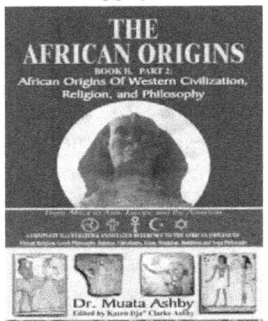

7. *AFRICAN ORIGINS BOOK 2 PART 2* African Origins of Western Civilization, Religion and Philosophy (Soft) -Soft Cover $24.95 ISBN: 1-884564-56-9

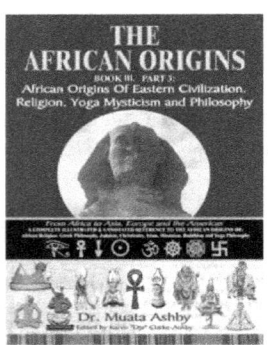

8. *EGYPT AND INDIA AFRICAN ORIGINS OF Eastern Civilization, Religion, Yoga Mysticism and Philosophy*-Soft Cover $29.95 (Soft) ISBN: 1-884564-57-7

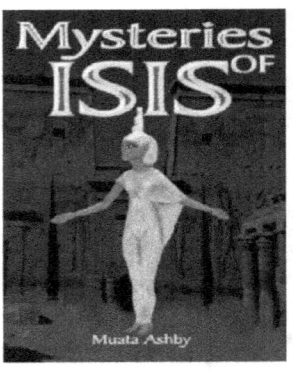

9. THE MYSTERIES OF ISIS: **The Ancient Egyptian Philosophy of Self-Realization** - There are several paths to discover the Divine and the mysteries of the higher Self. This volume details the mystery teachings of the goddess Aset (Isis) from Ancient Egypt- the path of wisdom. It includes the teachings of her temple and the disciplines that are enjoined for the initiates of the temple of Aset as they were given in ancient times. Also, this book includes the teachings of the main myths of Aset that lead a human being to spiritual enlightenment and immortality. Through the study of ancient myth and the illumination of initiatic understanding the idea of God is expanded from the mythological comprehension to the metaphysical. Then this metaphysical understanding is related to you, the student, so as to begin understanding your true divine nature. ISBN 1-884564-24-0 $22.99

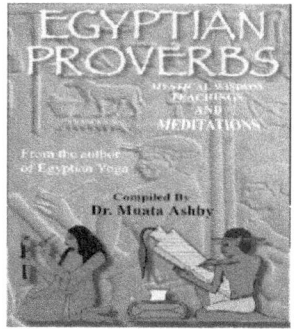

10. EGYPTIAN PROVERBS: collection of —Ancient Egyptian Proverbs and Wisdom Teachings -How to live according to MAAT Philosophy. Beginning Meditation. All proverbs are indexed for easy searches. For the first time in one volume, —— Ancient Egyptian Proverbs, wisdom teachings and meditations, fully illustrated with hieroglyphic text and symbols. EGYPTIAN PROVERBS is a unique collection of knowledge and wisdom which you can put into practice today and transform your life. $14.95 U.S   ISBN: 1-884564-00-3

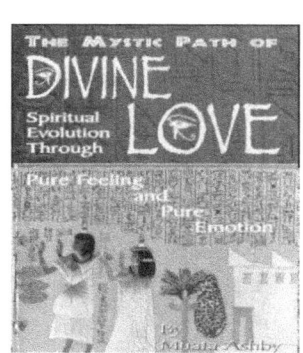

11. GOD OF LOVE: THE PATH OF DIVINE LOVE The Process of Mystical Transformation and The Path of Divine Love   This Volume focuses on the ancient wisdom teachings of "Neter Merri" –the Ancient Egyptian philosophy of Divine Love and how to use them in a scientific process for self-transformation. Love is one of the most powerful human emotions. It is also the source of Divine feeling that unifies God and the individual human being. When love is fragmented and diminished by egoism the Divine connection is lost. The Ancient tradition of Neter Merri leads human beings back to their Divine connection, allowing them to discover their innate glorious self that is actually Divine and immortal. This volume will detail the process of transformation from ordinary consciousness to cosmic consciousness through the integrated practice of the teachings and the path of Devotional Love toward the Divine. 5.5"x 8.5" ISBN 1-884564-11-9 $22.95

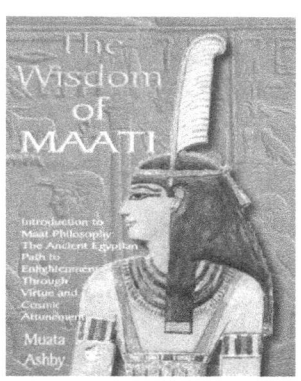

12. INTRODUCTION TO MAAT PHILOSOPHY: Spiritual Enlightenment Through the Path of Virtue Known commonly as Karma in India, the teachings of MAAT contain an extensive philosophy based on ariu (deeds) and their fructification in the form of shai and renenet (fortune and destiny, leading to Meskhenet (fate in a future birth) for living virtuously and with orderly wisdom are explained and the student is to begin practicing the precepts of Maat in daily life so as to promote the process of purification of the heart in preparation for the

judgment of the soul. This judgment will be understood not as an event that will occur at the time of death but as an event that occurs continuously, at every moment in the life of the individual. The student will learn how to become allied with the forces of the Higher Self and to thereby begin cleansing the mind (heart) of impurities so as to attain a higher vision of reality. ISBN 1-884564-20-8 $22.99

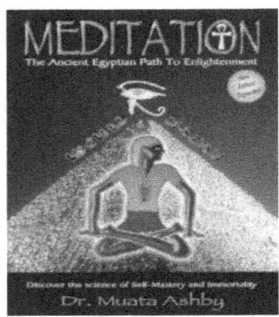

13. **MEDITATION The Ancient Egyptian Path to Enlightenment** Many people do not know about the rich history of meditation practice in Ancient Egypt. This volume outlines the theory of meditation and presents the Ancient Egyptian Hieroglyphic text which give instruction as to the nature of the mind and its three modes of expression. It also presents the texts which give instruction on the practice of meditation for spiritual Enlightenment and unity with the Divine. This volume allows the reader to begin practicing meditation by explaining, in easy to understand terms, the simplest form of meditation and working up to the most advanced form which was practiced in ancient times and which is still practiced by yogis around the world in modern times. ISBN 1-884564-27-7 $22.99

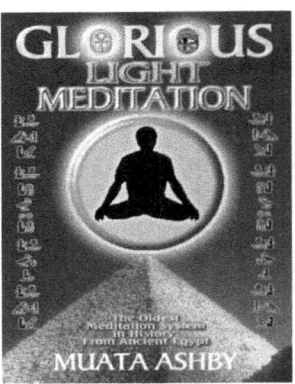

14. **THE GLORIOUS LIGHT MEDITATION TECHNIQUE OF ANCIENT EGYPT** New for the year 2000. This volume is based on the earliest known instruction in history given for the practice of formal meditation. Discovered by Dr. Muata Ashby, it is inscribed on the walls of the Tomb of Seti I in Thebes Egypt. This volume details the philosophy and practice of this unique system of meditation originated in Ancient Egypt and the earliest practice of meditation known in the world which occurred in the most advanced African Culture. ISBN: 1-884564-15-1 $16.95 (PB)

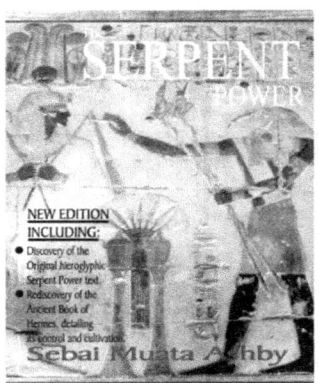

15. **THE SERPENT POWER: The Ancient Egyptian Mystical Wisdom of the Inner Life Force.** This Volume specifically deals with the latent life Force energy of the universe and in the human body, its control and

sublimation. How to develop the Life Force energy of the subtle body. This Volume will introduce the esoteric wisdom of the science of how virtuous living acts in a subtle and mysterious way to cleanse the latent psychic energy conduits and vortices of the spiritual body. ISBN 1-884564-19-4 $22.95

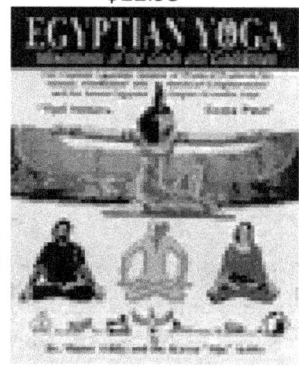

16. EGYPTIAN YOGA The Postures of The Gods and Goddesses Discover the physical postures and exercises practiced thousands of years ago in Ancient Egypt which are today known as Yoga exercises. Discover the history of the postures and how they were transferred from Ancient Egypt in Africa to India through Buddhist Tantrism. Then practice the postures as you discover the mythic teaching that originally gave birth to the postures and was practiced by the Ancient Egyptian priests and priestesses. This work is based on the pictures and teachings from the Creation story of Ra, The Asarian Resurrection Myth and the carvings and reliefs from various Temples in Ancient Egypt 8.5" X 11" ISBN 1-884564-10-0 Soft Cover $21.95 Exercise video $20

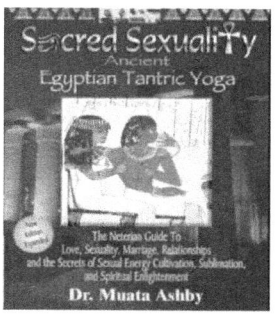

17. SACRED SEXUALITY: ANCIENT EGYPTIAN TANTRA YOGA: The Art of Sex Sublimation and Universal Consciousness This Volume will expand on the male and female principles within the human body and in the universe and further detail the sublimation of sexual energy into spiritual energy. The student will study the deities Min and Hathor, Asar and Aset, Geb and Nut and discover the mystical implications for a practical spiritual discipline. This Volume will also focus on the Tantric aspects of Ancient Egyptian and Indian mysticism, the purpose of sex and the mystical teachings of sexual sublimation which lead to self-knowledge and Enlightenment. ISBN 1-884564-03-8 $24.95

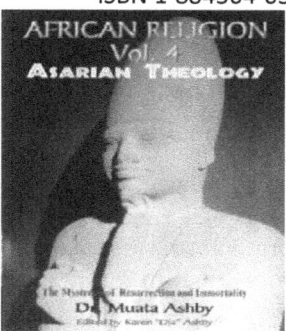

18. AFRICAN RELIGION Volume 4: ASARIAN THEOLOGY: RESURRECTING OSIRIS The path of Mystical Awakening and the Keys to Immortality NEW REVISED AND EXPANDED EDITION! The Ancient Sages created stories based on

human and superhuman beings whose struggles, aspirations, needs and desires ultimately lead them to discover their true Self. The myth of Aset, Asar and Heru is no exception in this area. While there is no one source where the entire story may be found, pieces of it are inscribed in various ancient Temples walls, tombs, steles and papyri. For the first time available, the complete myth of Asar, Aset and Heru has been compiled from original Ancient Egyptian, Greek and Coptic Texts. This epic myth has been richly illustrated with reliefs from the Temple of Heru at Edfu, the Temple of Aset at Philae, the Temple of Asar at Abydos, the Temple of Hathor at Denderah and various papyri, inscriptions and reliefs. Discover the myth which inspired the teachings of the *Shetaut Neter* (Egyptian Mystery System - Egyptian Yoga) and the Egyptian Book of Coming Forth By Day. Also, discover the three levels of Ancient Egyptian Religion, how to understand the mysteries of the Duat or Astral World and how to discover the abode of the Supreme in the Amenta, *The Other World* The ancient religion of Asar, Aset and Heru, if properly understood, contains all of the elements necessary to lead the sincere aspirant to attain immortality through inner self-discovery. This volume presents the entire myth and explores the main mystical themes and rituals associated with the myth for understating human existence, creation and the way to achieve spiritual emancipation - *Resurrection*. The Asarian myth is so powerful that it influenced and is still having an effect on the major world religions. Discover the origins and mystical meaning of the Christian Trinity, the Eucharist ritual and the ancient origin of the birthday of Jesus Christ. Soft Cover ISBN: 1-884564-27-5 $24.95

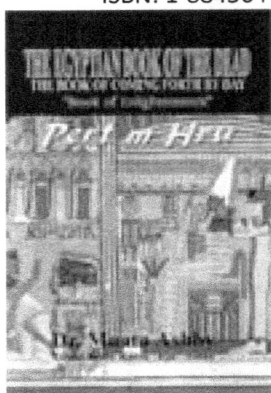

19. MYSTICISM OF THE PERT EM HERU

" I Know myself, I know myself, I am One With God!–From the Pert Em Heru "The Ru Pert em Heru" or "Ancient Egyptian Book of The Dead," or "Book of Coming Forth By Day" as it is more popularly known, has fascinated the world since the successful translation of Ancient Egyptian hieroglyphic scripture over 150 years ago. The astonishing writings in it reveal that the Ancient Egyptians believed in life after death and in an ultimate destiny to discover the Divine. The elegance and aesthetic beauty of the hieroglyphic text itself has inspired many see it as an art form in and of itself. But is there more to it than that? Did the Ancient Egyptian wisdom contain more than just aphorisms and hopes of eternal life beyond death? In this volume Dr. Muata Ashby, the author of over 25 books on Ancient Egyptian Yoga Philosophy has produced a new translation of the original texts which uncovers a mystical teaching underlying the sayings and rituals instituted by the Ancient Egyptian Sages and Saints. "Once the

philosophy of Ancient Egypt is understood as a mystical tradition instead of as a religion or primitive mythology, it reveals its secrets which if practiced today will lead anyone to discover the glory of spiritual self-discovery. The Pert em Heru is in every way comparable to the Indian Upanishads or the Tibetan Book of the Dead."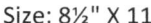
$28.95   ISBN# 1-884564-28-3
Size: 8½" X 11

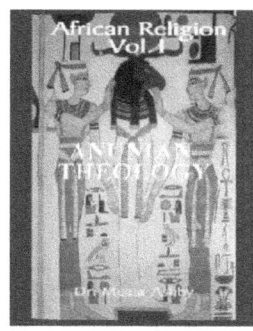

20. *African Religion VOL. 1- ANUNIAN THEOLOGY THE MYSTERIES OF RA* The Philosophy of Anu and The Mystical Teachings of The Ancient Egyptian Creation Myth Discover the mystical teachings contained in the Creation Myth and the gods and goddesses who brought creation and human beings into existence. The Creation myth of Anu is the source of Anunian Theology but also of the other main theological systems of Ancient Egypt that also influenced other world religions including Christianity, Hinduism and Buddhism. The Creation Myth holds the key to understanding the universe and for attaining spiritual Enlightenment. ISBN: 1-884564-38-0 $19.95

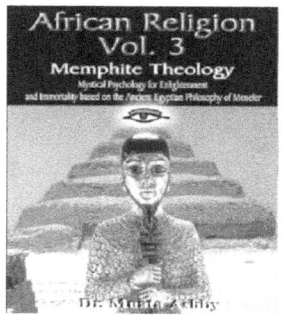

21. *African Religion VOL 3: Memphite Theology: MYSTERIES OF MIND* Mystical Psychology & Mental Health for Enlightenment and Immortality based on the Ancient Egyptian Philosophy of Menefer - Mysticism of Ptah, Egyptian Physics and Yoga Metaphysics and the Hidden properties of Matter. This volume uncovers the mystical psychology of the Ancient Egyptian wisdom teachings centering on the philosophy of the Ancient Egyptian city of Menefer (Memphite Theology). How to understand the mind and how to control the senses and lead the mind to health, clarity and mystical self-discovery. This Volume will also go deeper into the philosophy of God as creation and will explore the concepts of modern science and how they correlate with ancient teachings. This Volume will lay the ground work for the understanding of the philosophy of universal consciousness and the initiatic/yogic insight into who or what is God? ISBN 1-884564-07-0 $22.95

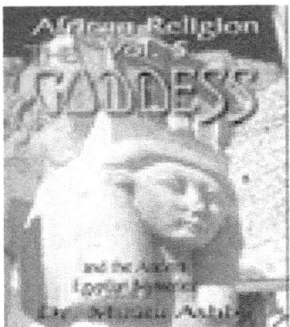

22. **AFRICAN RELIGION VOLUME 5: THE GODDESS AND THE EGYPTIAN MYSTERIESTHE PATH OF THE GODDESS THE GODDESS PATH** The Secret Forms of the Goddess and the Rituals of Resurrection The Supreme Being may be worshipped as father or as mother. *Ushet Rekhat* or *Mother Worship*, is the spiritual process of worshipping the Divine in the form of the Divine Goddess. It celebrates the most important forms of the Goddess including *Nathor, Maat, Aset, Arat, Amentet and Hathor* and explores their mystical meaning as well as the rising of *Sirius,* the star of Aset (Aset) and the new birth of Hor (Heru). The end of the year is a time of reckoning, reflection and engendering a new or renewed positive movement toward attaining spiritual Enlightenment. The Mother Worship devotional meditation ritual, performed on five days during the month of December and on New Year's Eve, is based on the Ushet Rekhit. During the ceremony, the cosmic forces, symbolized by Sirius - and the constellation of Orion ---, are harnessed through the understanding and devotional attitude of the participant. This propitiation draws the light of wisdom and health to all those who share in the ritual, leading to prosperity and wisdom. $14.95 ISBN 1-884564-18-6

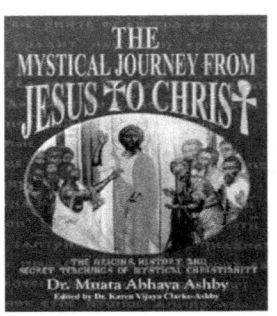

23. **THE MYSTICAL JOURNEY FROM JESUS TO CHRIST** Discover the ancient Egyptian origins of Christianity before the Catholic Church and learn the mystical teachings given by Jesus to assist all humanity in becoming Christlike. Discover the secret meaning of the Gospels that were discovered in Egypt. Also discover how and why so many Christian churches came into being. Discover that the Bible still holds the keys to mystical realization even though its original writings were changed by the church. Discover how to practice the original teachings of Christianity which leads to the Kingdom of Heaven. $24.95 ISBN# 1-884564-05-4 size: 8½" X 11"

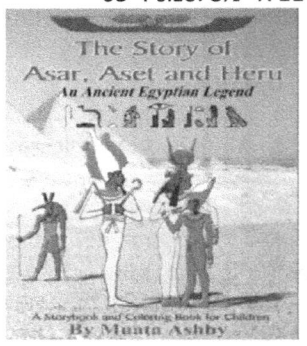

24. **THE STORY OF ASAR, ASET AND HERU:** An Ancient Egyptian Legend (For Children) Now for the first time, the most ancient myth of Ancient Egypt comes alive for

children. Inspired by the books *The Asarian Resurrection: The Ancient Egyptian Bible* and *The Mystical Teachings of The Asarian Resurrection, The Story of Asar, Aset and Heru* is an easy to understand and thrilling tale which inspired the children of Ancient Egypt to aspire to greatness and righteousness. If you and your child have enjoyed stories like *The Lion King* and *Star Wars* you will love *The Story of Asar, Aset and Heru*. Also, if you know the story of Jesus and Krishna you will discover than Ancient Egypt had a similar myth and that this myth carries important spiritual teachings for living a fruitful and fulfilling life. This book may be used along with *The Parents Guide To The Asarian Resurrection Myth: How to Teach Yourself and Your Child the Principles of Universal Mystical Religion*. The guide provides some background to the Asarian Resurrection myth and it also gives insight into the mystical teachings contained in it which you may introduce to your child. It is designed for parents who wish to grow spiritually with their children and it serves as an introduction for those who would like to study the Asarian Resurrection Myth in depth and to practice its teachings. 8.5" X 11"   ISBN: 1-884564-31-3 $12.95

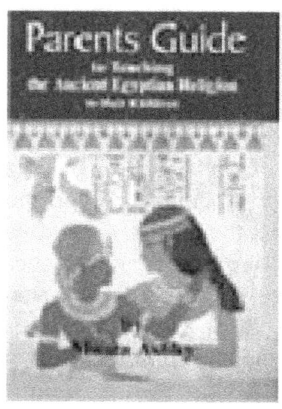

25. THE PARENTS GUIDE TO THE AUSARIAN RESURRECTION MYTH: How to Teach Yourself and Your Child the Principles of Universal Mystical Religion. This insightful manual brings for the timeless wisdom of the ancient through the Ancient Egyptian myth of Asar, Aset and Heru and the mystical teachings contained in it for parents who want to guide their children to understand and practice the teachings of mystical spirituality. This manual may be used with the children's storybook *The Story of Asar, Aset and Heru* by Dr. Muata Abhaya Ashby.   ISBN: 1-884564-30-5 $16.95

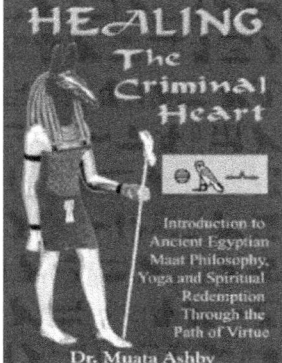

26. HEALING THE CRIMINAL HEART. Introduction to Maat Philosophy, Yoga and Spiritual Redemption Through the Path of Virtue   Who is a criminal? Is there such a thing as a

criminal heart? What is the source of evil and sinfulness and is there any way to rise above it? Is there redemption for those who have committed sins, even the worst crimes? Ancient Egyptian mystical psychology holds important answers to these questions. Over ten thousand years ago mystical psychologists, the Sages of Ancient Egypt, studied and charted the human mind and spirit and laid out a path which will lead to spiritual redemption, prosperity and Enlightenment. This introductory volume brings forth the teachings of the Asarian Resurrection, the most important myth of Ancient Egypt, with relation to the faults of human existence: anger, hatred, greed, lust, animosity, discontent, ignorance, egoism jealousy, bitterness, and a myriad of psycho-spiritual ailments which keep a human being in a state of negativity and adversity ISBN: 1-884564-17-8 $15.95

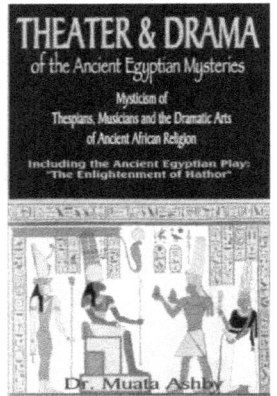

27. TEMPLE RITUAL OF THE ANCIENT EGYPTIAN MYSTERIES--THEATER & DRAMA OF THE ANCIENT EGYPTIAN MYSTERIES: Details the practice of the mysteries and ritual program of the temple and the philosophy an practice of the ritual of the mysteries, its purpose and execution. Featuring the Ancient Egyptian stage play-"The Enlightenment of Hathor' Based on an Ancient Egyptian Drama, The original Theater -Mysticism of the Temple of Hetheru 1-884564-14-3 $19.95 By Dr. Muata Ashby

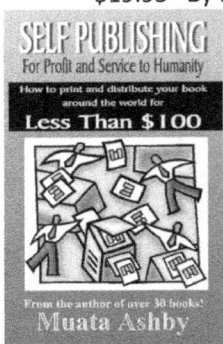

28. GUIDE TO PRINT ON DEMAND: SELF-PUBLISH FOR PROFIT, SPIRITUAL FULFILLMENT AND SERVICE TO HUMANITY Everyone asks us how we produced so many books in such a short time. Here are the secrets to writing and producing books that uplift humanity and how to get them printed for a fraction of the regular cost. Anyone can become an author even if they have limited funds. All that is necessary is the willingness to learn how the printing and book business work and the desire to follow the special instructions given here for preparing your manuscript format. Then you take your work directly to the non-traditional companies who can produce your books for less than the traditional book printer can. ISBN: 1-884564-40-2 $16.95 U. S.

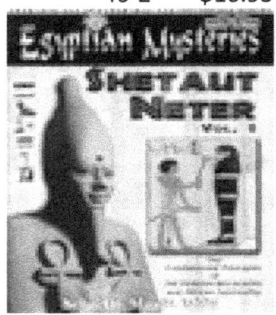

29. *Egyptian Mysteries: Vol. 1,* Shetaut Neter What are the Mysteries? For thousands of years the spiritual tradition of Ancient Egypt, *Shetaut Neter,* "The Egyptian Mysteries," "The Secret Teachings," have fascinated, tantalized and amazed the world. At one time exalted and recognized as the highest culture of the world, by Africans, Europeans, Asiatics, Hindus, Buddhists and other cultures of the ancient world, in time it was shunned by the emerging orthodox world religions. Its temples desecrated, its philosophy maligned, its tradition spurned, its philosophy dormant in the mystical *Medu Neter,* the mysterious hieroglyphic texts which hold the secret symbolic meaning that has scarcely been discerned up to now. What are the secrets of *Nehast* {spiritual awakening and emancipation, resurrection}. More than just a literal translation, this volume is for awakening to the secret code *Shetitu* of the teaching which was not deciphered by Egyptologists, nor could be understood by ordinary spiritualists. This book is a reinstatement of the original science made available for our times, to the reincarnated followers of Ancient Egyptian culture and the prospect of spiritual freedom to break the bonds of *Khemn,* "ignorance," and slavery to evil forces: *Sâaa* . ISBN: 1-884564-41-0 $19.99

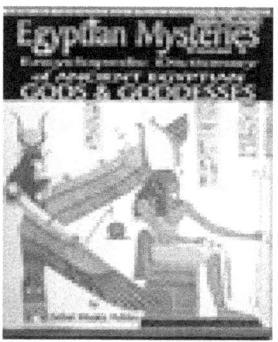

30. EGYPTIAN MYSTERIES VOL 2: Dictionary of Gods and Goddesses This book is about the mystery of neteru, the gods and goddesses of Ancient Egypt (Kamit, Kemet). Neteru means "Gods and Goddesses." But the Neterian teaching of Neteru represents more than the usual limited modern day concept of "divinities" or "spirits." The Neteru of Kamit are also metaphors, cosmic principles and vehicles for the enlightening teachings of Shetaut Neter (Ancient Egyptian-African Religion). Actually they are the elements for one of the most advanced systems of spirituality ever conceived in human history. Understanding the concept of neteru provides a firm basis for spiritual evolution and the pathway for viable culture, peace on earth and a healthy human society. Why is it important to have gods and goddesses in our lives? In order for spiritual evolution to be possible, once a human being has accepted that there is existence after death and there is a transcendental being who exists beyond time and space knowledge, human beings need a connection to that which transcends the ordinary experience of human life in time and space and a means to understand the transcendental reality beyond the mundane reality. ISBN: 1-884564-23-2 $21.95

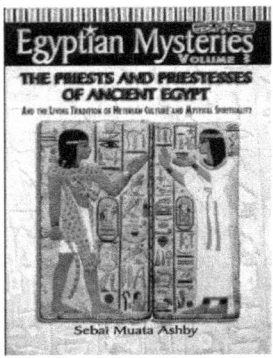

31. *EGYPTIAN MYSTERIES VOL. 3 The Priests and Priestesses of Ancient Egypt* This volume details the path of Neterian priesthood, the joys, challenges and rewards of advanced Neterian life, the teachings that allowed the priests and priestesses to manage the most long lived civilization in human history and how that path can be adopted today; for those who want to tread the path of the Clergy of Shetaut Neter. ISBN: 1-884564-53-4 $24.95

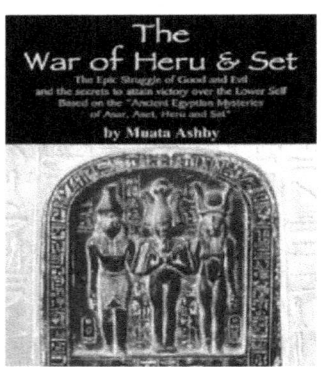

32. *The War of Heru and Set:* The Struggle of Good and Evil for Control of the World and The Human Soul This volume contains a novelized version of the Asarian Resurrection myth that is based on the actual scriptures presented in the Book Asarian Religion (old name – Resurrecting Osiris). This volume is prepared in the form of a screenplay and can be easily adapted to be used as a stage play. Spiritual seeking is a mythic journey that has many emotional highs and lows, ecstasies and depressions, victories and frustrations. This is the War of Life that is played out in the myth as the struggle of Heru and Set and those are mythic characters that represent the human Higher and Lower self. How to understand the war and emerge victorious in the journey o life? The ultimate victory and fulfillment can be experienced, which is not changeable or lost in time. The purpose of myth is to convey the wisdom of life through the story of divinities who show the way to overcome the challenges and foibles of life. In this volume the feelings and emotions of the characters of the myth have been highlighted to show the deeply rich texture of the Ancient Egyptian myth. This myth contains deep spiritual teachings and insights into the nature of self, of God and the mysteries of life and the means to discover the true meaning of life and thereby achieve the true purpose of life. To become victorious in the battle of life means to become the King (or Queen) of Egypt. Have you seen movies like The Lion King, Hamlet, The Odyssey, or The Little Buddha? These have been some of the most popular movies in modern times. The Sema Institute of Yoga is dedicated to researching and presenting the wisdom and culture of ancient Africa. The Script is designed to be produced as a motion picture but may be addapted for the theater as well. $21.95 copyright 1998 By Dr. Muata Ashby ISBN 1-8840564-44-5

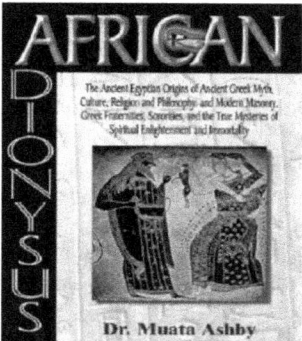

33. *AFRICAN DIONYSUS: FROM EGYPT TO GREECE:* The Kamitan Origins of Greek Culture and Religion ISBN: 1-884564-47-X FROM EGYPT TO GREECE This insightful manual is a reference to Ancient Egyptian mythology and philosophy and its correlation to what later became known as Greek and Rome mythology and philosophy. It outlines the basic tenets of the mythologies and shoes the ancient origins of Greek culture in Ancient Egypt. This volume also documents the origins of the Greek alphabet in Egypt as well as Greek religion, myth and philosophy of the gods and goddesses from Egypt from the myth of Atlantis and archaic period with the Minoans to the Classical period. This volume also acts as a resource for Colleges students who would like to set up fraternities and sororities based on the original Ancient Egyptian principles of Sheti and Maat philosophy. ISBN: 1-884564-47-X $22.95 U.S.

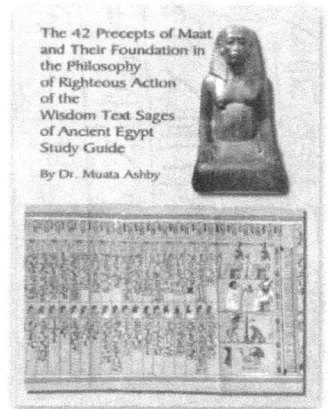

34. THE FORTY TWO PRECEPTS OF MAAT, THE PHILOSOPHY OF RIGHTEOUS ACTION AND THE ANCIENT EGYPTIAN WISDOM TEXTS ADVANCED STUDIES This manual is designed for use with the 1998 Maat Philosophy Class conducted by Dr. Muata Ashby. This is a detailed study of Maat Philosophy. It contains a compilation of the 42 laws or precepts of Maat and the corresponding principles which they represent along with the teachings of the ancient Egyptian Sages relating to each. Maat philosophy was the basis of Ancient Egyptian society and government as well as the heart of Ancient Egyptian myth and spirituality. Maat is at once a goddess, a cosmic force and a living social doctrine, which promotes social harmony and thereby paves the way for spiritual evolution in all levels of society. ISBN: 1-884564-48-8 $16.95 U.S.

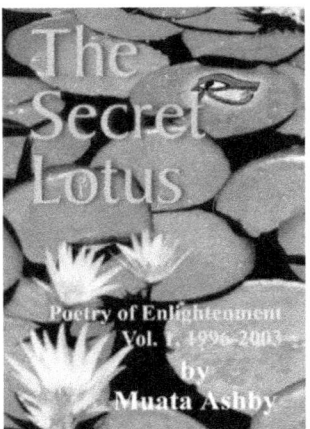

35. THE SECRET LOTUS: Poetry of Enlightenment

Discover the mystical sentiment of the Kemetic teaching as expressed through the poetry of Sebai Muata Ashby. The teaching of spiritual awakening is uniquely experienced when the poetic sensibility is present. This first volume contains the poems written between 1996 and 2003. **1-884564--16 -X $16.99**

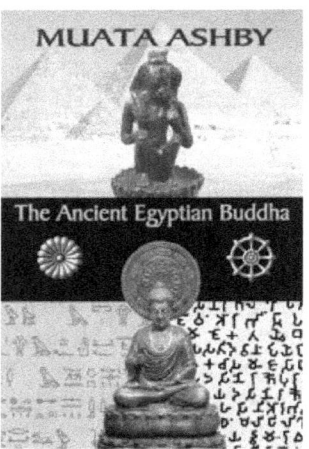

36. The Ancient Egyptian Buddha: The Ancient Egyptian Origins of Buddhism

This book is a compilation of several sections of a larger work, a book by the name of African Origins of Civilization, Religion, Yoga Mysticism and Ethics Philosophy. It also contains some additional evidences not contained in the larger work that demonstrate the correlation between Ancient Egyptian Religion and Buddhism. This book is one of several compiled short volumes that has been compiled so as to facilitate access to specific subjects contained in the larger work which is over 680 pages long. These short and small volumes have been specifically designed to cover one subject in a brief and low cost format. This present volume, The Ancient Egyptian Buddha: The Ancient Egyptian Origins of Buddhism, formed one subject in the larger work; actually it was one chapter of the larger work. However, this volume has some new additional evidences and comparisons of Buddhist and Neterian (Ancient Egyptian) philosophies not previously discussed. It was felt that this subject needed to be discussed because even in the early 21st century, the idea persists that Buddhism originated only in India independently. Yet there is ample evidence from ancient writings and perhaps more importantly, iconographical evidences from the Ancient Egyptians and early Buddhists themselves that prove otherwise. This handy volume has been designed to be accessible to young adults and all others who would like to have an easy reference with documentation on this important subject. This is an important subject because the frame of reference with which we look at a culture depends strongly on our conceptions about its origins. in this case, if we look at the Buddhism as an Asiatic religion we would treat it and it's culture in one way. If we id as African [Ancient Egyptian] we not only would see it in a different light but we also must ascribe Africa with a glorious legacy that matches any other culture in human history and gave rise to one of the present day most important religious philosophies. We would also look at the culture and philosophies of the Ancient Egyptians as having African insights that offer us greater depth into the Buddhist philosophies. Those insights inform our knowledge about other African traditions and we can also begin to understand in a deeper way the effect of Ancient Egyptian culture on African culture and also on the Asiatic as well. We would also be able to discover the glorious and wondrous teaching of mystical philosophy that Ancient Egyptian Shetaut Neter religion offers, that is as powerful as any other mystic system of spiritual philosophy in the world today. ISBN: 1-884564-61-5 $28.95

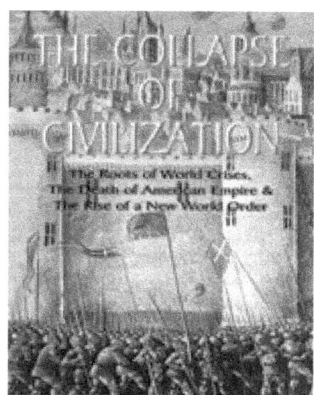

37. The Death of American Empire: Neo-conservatism, Theocracy, Economic Imperialism, Environmental Disaster and the Collapse of Civilization

This work is a collection of essays relating to social and economic, leadership, and ethics, ecological and religious issues that are facing the world today in order to understand the course of history that has led humanity to its present condition and then arrive at positive solutions that will lead to better outcomes for all humanity. It surveys the development and decline of major empires throughout history and focuses on the creation of American Empire along with the social, political and economic policies that led to the prominence of the United States of America as a Superpower including the rise of the political control of the neo-con political philosophy including militarism and the military industrial complex in American politics and the rise of the religious right into and American Theocracy movement. This volume details, through historical and current events, the psychology behind the dominance of western culture in world politics through the "Superpower Syndrome Mandatory Conflict Complex" that drives the Superpower culture to establish itself above all others and then act hubristically to dominate world culture through legitimate influences as well as coercion, media censorship and misinformation leading to international hegemony and world conflict. This volume also details the financial policies that gave rise to American prominence in the global economy, especially after World War II, and promoted American preeminence over the world economy through Globalization as well as the environmental policies, including the oil economy, that are promoting degradation of the world ecology and contribute to the decline of America as an Empire culture. This volume finally explores the factors pointing to the decline of the American Empire economy and imperial power and what to expect in the aftermath of American prominence and how to survive the decline while at the same time promoting policies and social-economic-religious-political changes that are needed in order to promote the emergence of a beneficial and sustainable culture. **$25.95soft** 1-884564-25-9, Hard Cover **$29.95** 1-884564-45-3

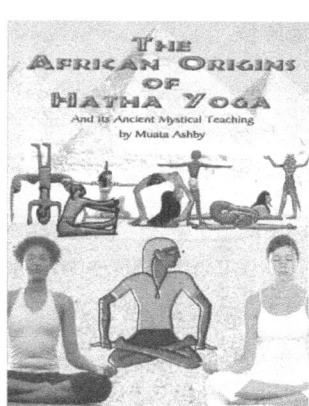

38. The African Origins of Hatha Yoga: And its Ancient Mystical Teaching

The subject of this present volume, The Ancient Egyptian Origins of Yoga Postures, formed one subject in the larger works, African Origins of Civilization Religion, Yoga Mysticism and Ethics Philosophy and the Book Egypt and India is the section of the book African Origins of Civilization. Those works contain the collection of all correlations between Ancient Egypt and India. This volume also contains some additional information not contained in the previous work. It was felt that this subject needed to be discussed more directly, being treated in one volume, as opposed to being contained in the larger work along with other subjects, because even in the early 21st century, the idea persists that the Yoga and specifically, Yoga Postures, were invented and developed only in India. The Ancient Egyptians were peoples originally from Africa who were, in ancient times, colonists in India. Therefore it is no surprise that many Indian traditions including religious and Yogic, would be found earlier in Ancient Egypt. Yet there is ample evidence from ancient writings and perhaps more importantly, iconographical evidences from the Ancient Egyptians themselves and the Indians themselves that prove the connection between Ancient Egypt and India as well as the existence of a discipline of Yoga Postures in Ancient Egypt long before its practice in India. This handy volume has been designed to be accessible to young adults and all others who would like to have an easy reference with documentation on this important subject. This is an important subject because the frame of reference with which we look at a culture depends strongly on our conceptions about its origins. In this case, if we look at the Ancient Egyptians as Asiatic peoples we would treat them and their culture in one way. If we see them as Africans we not only see them in a different light but we also must ascribe Africa with a glorious legacy that matches any other culture in human history. We would also look at the culture and philosophies of the Ancient Egyptians as having African insights instead of Asiatic ones. Those insights inform our knowledge bout other African traditions and we can also begin to understand in a deeper way the effect of Ancient Egyptian culture on African culture and also on the Asiatic as well. When we discover the deeper and more ancient practice of the postures system in Ancient Egypt that was called "Hatha Yoga" in India, we are able to find a new and expanded understanding of the practice that constitutes a discipline of spiritual practice that informs and revitalizes the Indian practices as well as all spiritual disciplines. $19.99 ISBN 1-884564-60-7

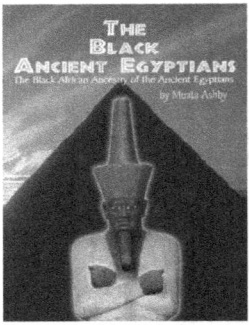

39. The Black Ancient Egyptians

This present volume, The Black Ancient Egyptians: The Black African Ancestry of the Ancient Egyptians, formed one subject in the larger work: The African Origins of Civilization, Religion, Yoga Mysticism and Ethics Philosophy. It was felt that this subject needed to be discussed because even in the early 21st century, the idea persists that the Ancient Egyptians were peoples originally from Asia Minor who came into North-East Africa. Yet there is ample evidence from ancient writings and perhaps more importantly, iconographical evidences from the Ancient Egyptians themselves that proves otherwise. This handy volume has been designed to be accessible to young adults and all others who would like to have an easy reference with documentation on this important subject. This is an important subject because the frame of reference with which we look at a culture depends strongly on our conceptions about its origins. in this case, if we look at the Ancient Egyptians as Asiatic peoples we would treat them and their culture in one way. If we see them as Africans we not only see them in a different light but we also must ascribe Africa with a glorious legacy that matches any other culture in human history. We would also look at the culture and philosophies of the Ancient Egyptians as having African insights instead of Asiatic ones. Those insights inform our knowledge bout other African traditions and we can also begin to understand in a deeper way the effect of Ancient Egyptian culture on African culture and also on the Asiatic as well. ISBN 1-884564-21-6 $19.99

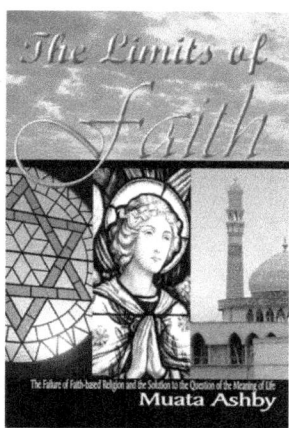

40. The Limits of Faith: The Failure of Faith-based Religions and the Solution to the Meaning of Life

Is faith belief in something without proof? And if so is there never to be any proof or discovery? If so what is the need of intellect? If faith is trust in something that is real is that reality historical, literal or metaphorical or philosophical? If knowledge is an essential element in faith why should there by so much emphasis on believing and not on understanding in the modern practice of religion? This volume is a compilation of essays related to the nature of religious faith in the context of its inception in human history as well as its meaning for religious practice and relations between religions in modern times. Faith has come to be regarded as a virtuous goal in life. However, many people have asked how can it be that an endeavor that is supposed to be dedicated to spiritual upliftment has led to more conflict in human history than any other social factor? ISBN 1884564631 SOFT COVER - $19.99, ISBN 1884564623 HARD COVER -$28.95

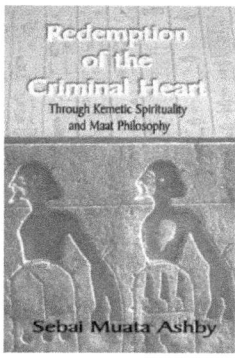

41. Redemption of The Criminal Heart Through Kemetic Spirituality and Maat Philosophy

Special book dedicated to inmates, their families and members of the Law Enforcement community. ISBN: 1-884564-70-4
$5.00

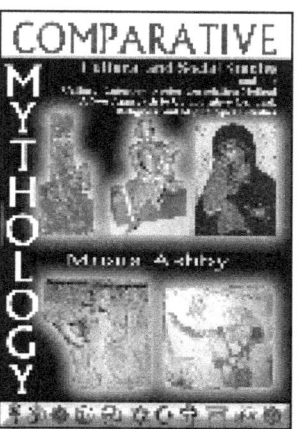

42. COMPARATIVE MYTHOLOGY

What are Myth and Culture and what is their importance for understanding the development of societies, human evolution and the search for meaning? What is the purpose of culture and how do cultures evolve? What are the elements of a culture and how can those elements be broken down and the constituent parts of a culture understood and compared? How do cultures interact? How does enculturation occur and how do people interact with other cultures? How do the processes of acculturation and cooptation occur and what does this mean for the development of a society? How can the study of myths and the elements of culture help in understanding the meaning of life and the means to promote understanding and peace in the world of human activity? This volume is the exposition of a method for studying and comparing cultures, myths and other social aspects of a society. It is an expansion on the Cultural Category Factor Correlation method for studying and comparing myths, cultures, religions and other aspects of human culture. It was originally introduced in the year 2002. This volume contains an expanded treatment as well as several refinements along with examples of the application of the method. the apparent. I hope you enjoy these art renditions as serene reflections of the mysteries of life. ISBN: 1-884564-72-0 Book price $21.95

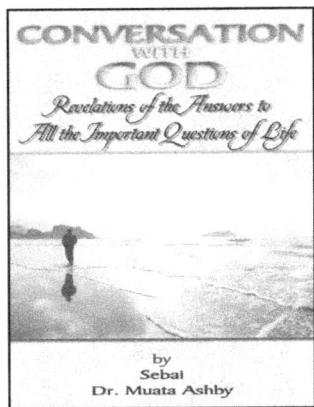

43. CONVERSATION WITH GOD: Revelations of the Important Questions of Life
$24.99 U.S.

This volume contains a grouping of some of the questions that have been submitted to Sebai Dr. Muata Ashby. They are efforts by many aspirants to better understand and practice the teachings of mystical spirituality. It is said that when sages are asked spiritual questions they are relaying the wisdom of God, the Goddess, the Higher Self, etc. There is a very special quality about the Q & A process that does not occur during a regular lecture session. Certain points come out that would not come out otherwise due to the nature of the process which ideally occurs after a lecture. Having been to a certain degree enlightened by a lecture certain new questions arise and the answers to these have the effect of elevating the teaching of the lecture to even higher levels. Therefore, enjoy these exchanges and may they lead you to enlightenment, peace and prosperity. Available Late Summer 2007 ISBN: 1-884564-68-2

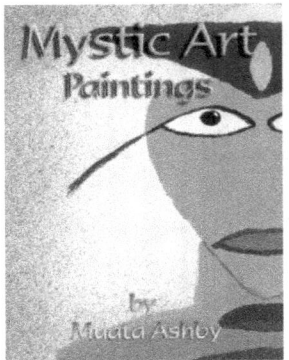

44. MYSTIC ART PAINTINGS
(with Full Color images) This book contains a collection of the small number of paintings that I have created over the years. Some were used as early book covers and others were done simply to express certain spiritual feelings; some were created for no purpose except to express the joy of color and the feeling of relaxed freedom. All are to elicit mystical awakening in the viewer. Writing a book on philosophy is like sculpture, the more the work is rewritten the reflections and ideas become honed and take form and become clearer and imbued with intellectual beauty. Mystic music is like meditation, a world of its own that exists about 1 inch above ground wherein the musician does not touch the ground. Mystic Graphic Art is meditation in form, color, image and reflected image which opens the door to the reality behind the apparent. I hope you enjoy these art renditions and my reflections on them as serene reflections of the mysteries of life, as visual renditions of the philosophy I have written about over the years. ISBN 1-884564-69-0 $19.95

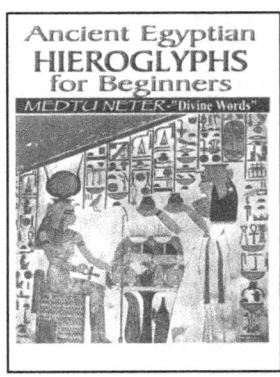

45. ANCIENT EGYPTIAN HIEROGLYPHS FOR BEGINNERS

This brief guide was prepared for those inquiring about how to enter into Hieroglyphic studies on their own at home or in study groups. First of all you should know that there are a few institutions around the world which teach how to read the Hieroglyphic text but due to the nature of the study there are perhaps only a handful of people who can read fluently. It is possible for anyone with average intelligence to achieve a high level of proficiency in reading inscriptions on temples and artifacts; however, reading extensive texts is another issue entirely. However, this introduction will give you entry into those texts if assisted by dictionaries and other aids. Most Egyptologists have a basic knowledge and keep dictionaries and notes handy when it comes to dealing with more difficult texts. Medtu Neter or the Ancient Egyptian hieroglyphic language has been considered as a "Dead Language." However, dead languages have always been studied by individuals who for the most part have taught themselves through various means. This book will discuss those means and how to use them most efficiently. ISBN 1884564429 **$28.95**

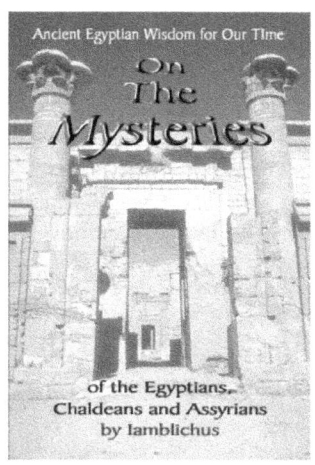

46. ON THE MYSTERIES: Wisdom of An Ancient Egyptian Sage -with Foreword by Muata Ashby

This volume, On the Mysteries, by Iamblichus (Abamun) is a unique form or scripture out of the Ancient Egyptian religious tradition. It is written in a form that is not usual or which is not usually found in the remnants of Ancient Egyptian scriptures. It is in the form of teacher and disciple, much like the Eastern scriptures such as Bhagavad Gita or the Upanishads. This form of writing may not have been necessary in Ancient times, because the format of teaching in Egypt was different prior to the conquest period by the Persians, Assyrians, Greeks and later the Romans. The question and answer format can be found but such extensive discourses and corrections of misunderstandings within the context of a teacher - disciple relationship is not usual. It therefore provides extensive insights into the times when it was written and the state of practice of Ancient Egyptian and other mystery religions. This has important implications for our times because we are today, as in the Greco-Roman period, also besieged with varied religions and new age philosophies as well as social strife and war. How can we understand our times and also make sense of the forest of spiritual traditions? How can we cut through the cacophony of religious fanaticism, and ignorance as well as misconceptions about the mysteries on the other in order to discover the true purpose of religion and the secret teachings that open up the mysteries of life and the way to enlightenment and immortality? This book, which comes to us from so long ago, offers us transcendental wisdom that applied to the world two thousand years ago as well as our world today. ISBN 1-884564-64-X **$25.95**

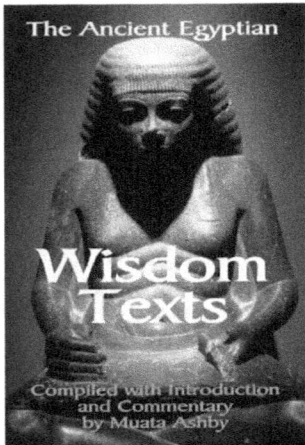

47. The Ancient Egyptian Wisdom Texts - Compiled by Muata Ashby
The Ancient Egyptian Wisdom Texts are a genre of writings from the ancient culture that have survived to the present and provide a vibrant record of the practice of spiritual evolution otherwise known as religion or yoga philosophy in Ancient Egypt. The principle focus of the Wisdom Texts is the cultivation of understanding, peace, harmony, selfless service, self-control, Inner fulfillment and spiritual realization. When these factors are cultivated in human life, the virtuous qualities in a human being begin to manifest and sinfulness, ignorance and negativity diminish until a person is able to enter into higher consciousness, the coveted goal of all civilizations. It is this virtuous mode of life which opens the door to self-discovery and spiritual enlightenment. Therefore, the Wisdom Texts are important scriptures on the subject of human nature, spiritual psychology and mystical philosophy. The teachings presented in the Wisdom Texts form the foundation of religion as well as the guidelines for conducting the affairs of every area of social interaction including commerce, education, the army, marriage, and especially the legal system. These texts were sources for the famous 42 Precepts of Maat of the Pert-m-Heru (Book of the Dead), essential regulations of good conduct to develop virtue and purity in order to attain higher consciousness and immortality after death. ISBN1-884564-65-8 $18.95

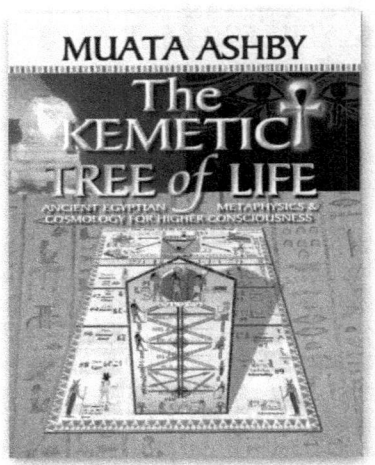

48. THE KEMETIC TREE OF LIFE
THE KEMETIC TREE OF LIFE: Newly Revealed Ancient Egyptian Cosmology and Metaphysics for Higher Consciousness The Tree of Life is a roadmap of a journey which explains how Creation came into being and how it will end. It also explains what Creation is composed of and also what human beings are and what they are composed of. It also explains the process of Creation, how Creation develops, as well as who created Creation and where that entity may be found. It also explains how a human being may discover that entity and in so doing also discover the secrets of Creation, the meaning of life and the means to break free from the pathetic condition of human limitation and mortality in order to discover the higher realms of being by discovering the principles, the levels of existence that are beyond the simple physical and material aspects of life. This book contains color plates   **ISBN: 1-884564-74-7**

$27.95 U.S.

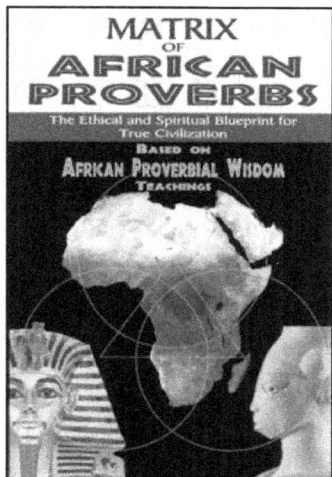

49-MATRIX OF AFRICAN PROVERBS: The Ethical and Spiritual Blueprint

This volume sets forth the fundamental principles of African ethics and their practical applications for use by individuals and organizations seeking to model their ethical policies using the Traditional African values and concepts of ethical human behavior for the proper sustenance and management of society. Furthermore, this book will provide guidance as to how the Traditional African Ethics may be viewed and applied, taking into consideration the technological and social advancements in the present. This volume also presents the principles of ethical culture, and references for each to specific injunctions from Traditional African Proverbial Wisdom Teachings. These teachings are compiled from varied Pre-colonial African societies including Yoruba, Ashanti, Kemet, Malawi, Nigeria, Ethiopia, Galla, Ghana and many more. ISBN 1-884564-77-1

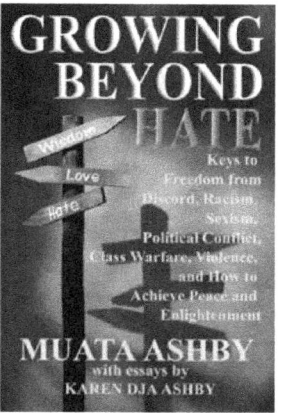

50- Growing Beyond Hate: Keys to Freedom from Discord, Racism, Sexism, Political Conflict, Class Warfare, Violence, and How to Achieve Peace and Enlightenment

---INTRODUCTION: WHY DO WE HATE? Hatred is one of the fundamental motivating aspects of human life; the other is desire. Desire can be of a worldly nature or of a spiritual, elevating nature. Worldly desire and hatred are like two sides of the same coin in that human life is usually swaying from one to the other; but the question is why? And is there a way to satisfy the desiring or hating mind in such a way as to find peace in life? Why do human beings go to war? Why do human beings perpetrate violence against one another? And is there a way not just to understand the phenomena but to resolve the issues that plague humanity and could lead to a more harmonious society? Hatred is perhaps the greatest scourge of humanity in that it leads to misunderstanding, conflict and untold miseries of life and clashes between individuals, societies and nations. Therefore, the riddle of Hatred, that is, understanding the sources of it and how to confront, reduce and even eradicate it so as to bring forth the fulfillment in life and peace for society, should be a top priority for social scientists, spiritualists and philosophers. This book is written from the perspective of spiritual philosophy based on the mystical wisdom and sema or yoga philosophy of the Ancient Egyptians. This philosophy, originated and based in the wisdom of Shetaut Neter, the Egyptian Mysteries, and Maat, ethical way of life in society and in spirit, contains

Sema-Yogic wisdom and understanding of life's predicaments that can allow a human being of any ethnic group to understand and overcome the causes of hatred, racism, sexism, violence and disharmony in life, that plague human society. ISBN: 1-884564-81-X

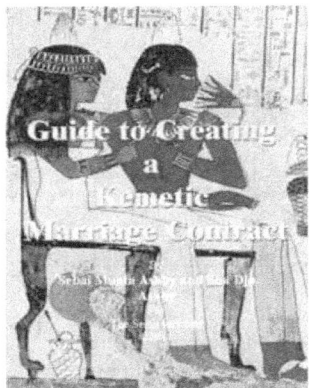

52. Guide to Creating a Kemetic Marriage Contract

This marital contract guide reflects actual Ancient Egyptian Principles for Kemetic Marriage as they are to be applied for our times. The marital contract allows people to have a framework with which to face the challenges of marital relations instead of relying on hopes or romantic dreams that everything will workout somehow; in other words, love is not all you need. The latter is not an evolved, mature way of handling one of the most important aspects of human life. Therefore, it behooves anyone who wishes to enter into a marriage to explore the issues, express their needs and seek to avoid costly mistakes, and resolve conflicts in the normal course of life or make sure that their rights and dignity will be protected if any eventuality should occur. Marital relations in Ancient Egypt were not like those in other countries of the time and not like those of present day countries. The extreme longevity of Ancient Egyptian society, founded in Maat philosophy, allowed the social development of marriage to evolve and progress to a high level of order and balance. Maat represents truth, righteous, justice and harmony in life. This meant that the marital partner's rights were to be protected with equal standing before the law. So there was no disparity between rights of men or rights of women. Therefore, anyone who wants to enter into a marriage based on Kemetic principles must first and foremost adhere to this standard…equality in the rights of men and women. This guide demonstrates procedures for following the Ancient Egyptian practice of formalizing marriage with a contract that spells out the important concerns of each partner in the marital relationship, based on Maatian principles [of righteous, truth, harmony and justice] so that the rights and needs of each partner may be protected within the marriage. It also allows the partners to think about issues that arise out of the marital relations so that they may have a foundation to fall back on in the event that those or other unforeseen issues arise and cause conflict in the relationship. By having a document of expressed concerns, needs and steps to be taken to address them, it is less likely that issues which affect the relationship in a negative way will arise, and when they do, they will be better handled, in a more balanced, just and amicable way.
EBOOK ISBN 978-1-937016-59-3, HARDCOPY BOOK ISBN: 1-884564-82-8

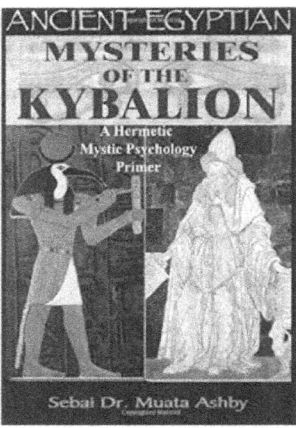

53-Ancient Egyptian Mysteries of The Kybalion: A Hermetic Mystic Psychology Primer Paperback – November 28, 2014

This Volume is a landmark study by a renounced mystic philosopher, Sebai Dr.

Muata Ashby. It is study not just to philosophize but to be practiced for the purpose of attaining enlightenment. The book is divided into three sections. Part 1 INTRODUCTION presents a brief history of Hermeticism, its origins in the Ancient Egyptian Mysteries (Neterianism) the Kybalion and the origins of the personality known as Hermes Trismegistus. Part 2 presents the essential teachings of the Kybalion text, a set of MAXIMS, without interpretation. Part 3 presents glosses (commentary and explanation) on the essential teachings of the Kybalion based on the philosophy of the Ancient Egyptian Mysteries as determined by Sebai Dr. Muata Ashby based on studies and translations of original Ancient Egyptian Hieroglyphic texts; the source from which the Kybalion teaching is derived. The Glosses are an edited and expanded version of Lessons given by Sebai Dr. Muata Ashby in the form of lectures on the teachings of the Kybalion.

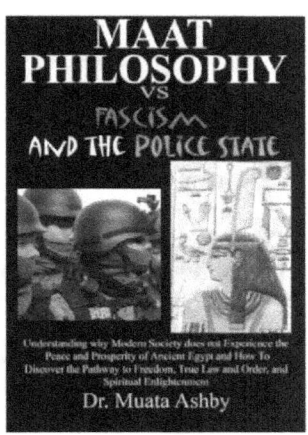

54-Maat Philosophy Versus Fascism and the Police State: Understanding why Modern Society does not Experience the Peace and Prosperity of Ancient Egypt ... Law and Order, and Spiritual Enlightenment Paperback – January 1, 2014

Understanding why Modern Society does not Experience the Peace and Prosperity of Ancient Egypt and How To Discover the Pathway to Freedom, True Law and Order, and Spiritual Enlightenment. Understanding the Corporate State and How Maatian Philosophy can Leads to Freedom, Prosperity and Enlightenment

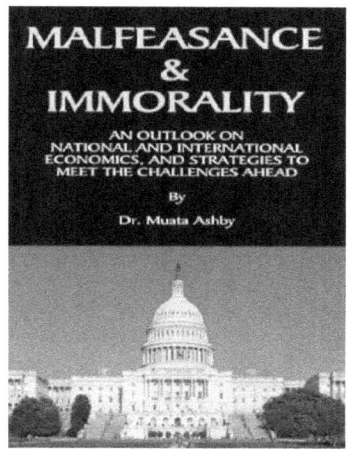

55- MALFEASANCE & IMMORALITY: An Analysis of the World Economic Crash of 2008, the Corrupt Political and Financial Institutions that Caused it and Strategies to Survive the Future Collapse of the Economy

The following is a first ever publication, by the Sema Institute, of a ◆White Paper◆. The term is defined as: A white paper is an authoritative report or guide that often addresses issues and how to solve them. White papers are used to educate readers and help people make decisions. They are often used in politics and business. This paper serves as an update to the book Dollar Crisis: The Collapse of Society and Redemption Through Ancient Egyptian Fiscal & Monetary Policy (2008). That book was a continuation and expansion of issues presented in the book The Collapse of Civilization and the Death of American Empire (2006). Those books contained a detailed analysis of economic and political as well as social issues and how Maat Philosophy could offer insights into the nature of the problem, its sources and possible solutions as well as a means to develop an economic system (Fiscal and Monetary policies) that can work for all members of society. This paper contains an analysis of economic events and possible future outcomes based on those events as well as ideas individuals or groups may use in order to develop plans of action to deal with the possible detrimental events that may occur in the near and intermediate future. It serves as an update to the previous publications. This paper is divided into two parts. The first section is a summary which contains the conclusions of each section of Part 2. This was done so that the reader may have a quick and easy understanding of what is happening with the economy and finally, the actions that should be considered to meet the challenges ahead

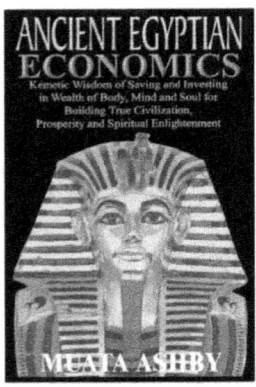

56- ANCIENT EGYPTIAN ECONOMICS
Ancient Egyptian Economics: Kemetic Wisdom of Saving and Investing in Wealth of Body, Mind and Soul for Building True Civilization, Prosperity and Spiritual Enlightenment------Question: Why has the subject of finances and economics become important, I thought the spiritual teachings and Ancient Egyptian Philosophy and money were separate? Answer: Finances and money are an integral part of Ancient Egyptian culture as an instrument for promoting Maat ethics in the form of the well-being of the 'hekat'. The hekat are the people and the "Heka" is the Pharaoh. The Pharaoh was like a shepherd leading a flock and moneys were controlled righteously to promote the welfare of the people. In that tradition we have applied the philosophy of maatian economics to promote the well-being of those who are following this path as well as those who may read the books so they may avoid financial trouble as much as possible and have better capacity to practice the teachings. In order to have a successful life, human beings need a certain amount of money and wealth, but money and wealth are not the goal. They are a foundation that enables the true goal of life, enlightenment, to be realized. Therefore, we are only fulfilling the duty of transmitting wisdom about wealth to promote Maat, righteousness, truth and well-being, for all. This volume explores the mysteries of wealth based on the teachings of the sages of Ancient Egypt and the means to promote prosperity that allows a person to create the conditions for discovering inner peace and spiritual enlightenment. HTP-Peace

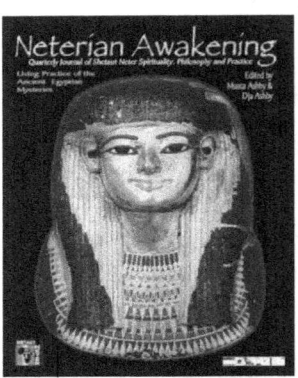

57- NETERIAN AWAKENING Journal of Neterian Culture Vol 1-12 In one Volume

This is a single file containing 12 volumes of The Neterian Awakening Journal. The Neterian Awakening Journal was a publication where the culture and community of Shetaut Neter spirituality was explored. In it Sebai Dr. Muata Ashby and Dr. Dja Ashby along with members of the Temple of Shetaut Neter presented articles, festival reviews, Questions and Answer columns and many other important aspects of Neterian culture and spirituality beyond those presented in other volumes of the book series that are useful in understanding the practice of Neterian Spirituality and the path to achieving a ◆Neterian Spiritual Awakening.◆ Part of its mission was: To promote the study of Shetaut Neter (Neterianism, Neterian Religion) as a spiritual path. Instruct the serious followers of Shetaut Neter spirituality who would like to receive literature in between the publication of major books that will fill the needs of their daily spiritual practice. Neterian Awakening Journal explores the varied aspects of Shetaut Neter spirituality not covered in the books. NAJ provides a forum for the development of a Neterian Community of those who wish to follow the Neterian Spiritual Path of African Religious Culture

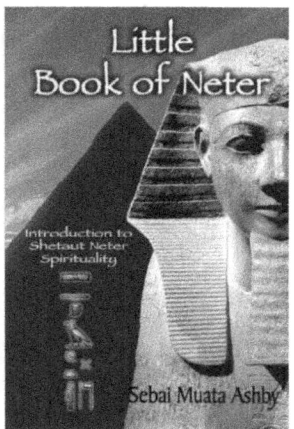

58- Little Book of Neter: Introduction to Shetaut Neter Spirituality and Religion Paperback – June 7, 2007

The Little Book of Neter is a summary of the most important teachings of Shetaut Neter for all aspirants to have for easy reference and distribution. It is designed to be portable and low cost so that all can have the main teachings of Shetaut Neter at easy access for personal use and also for sharing with others the basic tenets of Neterian spirituality.

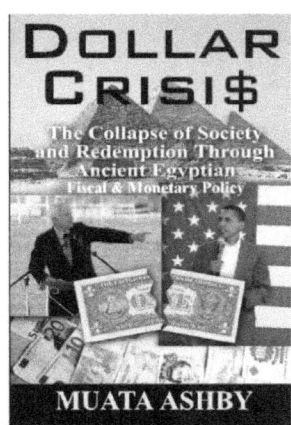

59- Dollar Crisis: The Collapse of Society and Redemption Through Ancient Egyptian Monetary Policy by Muata Ashby (2008-07-24)

This book is about the problems of the US economy and the imminent collapse of the U.S. Dollar and its dire consequences for the US economy and the world. It is also about the corruption in government, economics and social order that led to this point. Also it is about survival, how to make it through this perhaps most trying period in the history of the United States. Also it is about the ancient wisdom of life that allowed an ancient civilization to grow beyond the destructive corruptions of ignorance and power so that the people of today may gain insight into the nature of their condition, how they got there and what needs to be done in order to salvage what is left and rebuild a society that is sustainable, beneficial and an example for all humanity.

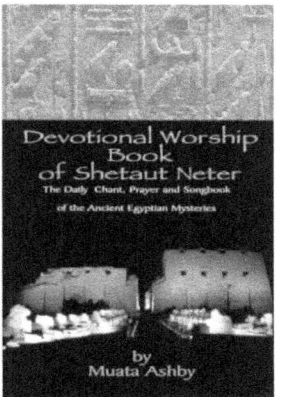

60- Devotional Worship Book of Shetaut Neter: Medu Neter song, chant and hymn book for daily practice [Paperback] [2007] (Author) Muata Ashby Paperback – 2007

Ushet Hekau Shedi Sema Taui Uashu or Ushet means "to worship the Divine," "to propitiate the Divine." Ushet is of two types, external and internal. When you go to pilgrimage centers, temples, spiritual gatherings, etc., you are practicing external worship or spiritual practice. When you go into your private meditation room on your own and your utter words of power, prayers and meditation you are practicing internal worship or spiritual practice. Ushet needs to be understood as a process of not only an outer show of spiritual practice, but it is also a process of developing love for the Divine. Therefore, Ushet really signifies a development in Devotion towards the Divine. This practice is also known as sma uash or Yoga of Devotion. Ushet is the process of discovering the Divine and allowing your heart to flow towards the Divine. This program of life allows a spiritual aspirant to develop inner peace, contentment and universal love, and these qualities lead to spiritual enlightenment or union with the Divine. It is recommended that you see the book "The Path of Divine Love" by Dr. Muata Ashby. This volume will give details into this form of Sema or Yoga.

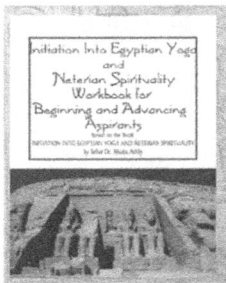

61- Initiation Into Egyptian Yoga and Neterian Religion Workbook for Beginning and Advancing Aspirants

What is Initiation? The great personalities of the past known to the world as Isis, Hathor, Jesus, Buddha and many other great Sages and Saints were initiated into their spiritual path but how did initiation help them and what were they specifically initiated into? This volume is a template for such lofty studies, a guidebook and blueprint for aspirants who want to understand what the path is all about, its requirements and goals, as they work with a qualified spiritual guide as they tread the path of Kemetic Spirituality and Yoga disciplines. This workbook helps by presenting the fundamental teachings of Egyptian Yoga and Neterian Spirituality with questions and exercises to help the aspirant gain a foundation for more advanced studies and practices

HIEROGLYPH TRANSLATION SERIES BY
Dr. Muata Ashby

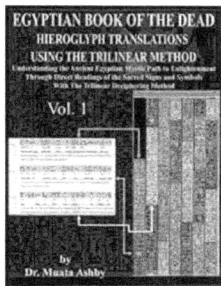

Egyptian Book of the Dead Hieroglyph Translations Using the Trilinear Method: Understanding th Mystic Path to Enlightenment...

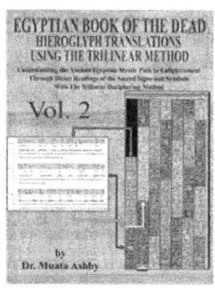

Egyptian Book of the Dead Hieroglyph Translations Using The Trilinear Method Vol. 2: Understanding the Mystic Path to...
by Muata Ashby

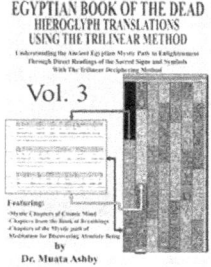

EGYPTIAN BOOK OF THE DEAD HIEROGLYPH TRANSLATIONS USING THE TRILINEAR METHOD Volume 3: Understanding the Mystic Path to...
by Muata Ashby

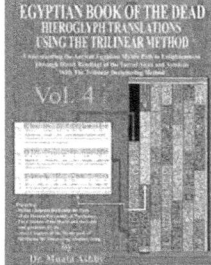

EGYPTIAN BOOK OF THE DEAD HIEROGLYPH TRANSLATIONS USING THE TRILINEAR METHOD Volume 4: Understanding the Mystic Path to...

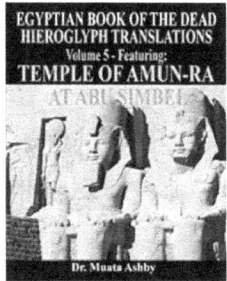

EGYPTIAN BOOK OF THE DEAD HIEROGLYPH TRANSLATIONS USING THE TRILINEAR METHOD Volume 5: Featuring Temple of Amun-Ra at Ab...
by Muata Ashby

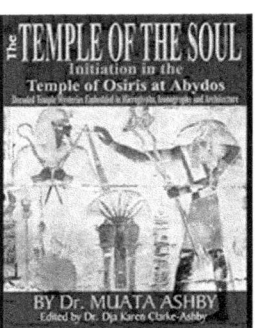
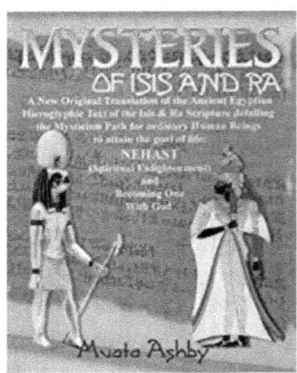

Temple of the Soul Initiation Philosophy in the Temple of Osiris at Abydos: Decoded Temple Mysteries Translations of Temple Inscriptions...
by Muata Ashby

Mysteries of Isis and Ra: A New Original Translation Hieroglyphic Scripture of t
by Muata Ashby

www.ingramcontent.com/pod-product-compliance
Lightning Source LLC
Chambersburg PA
CBHW081742100526
44592CB00015B/2269